D1824514

Bacterial Toxins

Series editors

Dr J A Cole, University of Birmingham
Dr C J Knowles, University of Kent

Titles in series

Oral Microbiology   *P Marsh*

Bacterial Toxins   *J Stephen and R A Pietrowski*

The Microbial Cell Cycle   *C Edwards*

Bacterial Plasmids   *K Hardy*

Extrachromosomal Inheritance   *S Oliver*

Respiratory Chain and Photosynthetic Energy Conservation in Bacteria   *C W Jones*

Spore Formation in Bacteria   *A Moir*

The Structure of the Bacterial Cell   *H J Rogers*

Aspects of Microbiology

Bacterial Toxins

J. Stephen
Senior Lecturer, Department of Microbiology, University of Birmingham

R. A. Pietrowski
Senior Bacteriologist in Vaccines Research and Development
Glaxo Operations UK Ltd, Speke, Liverpool.

Nelson

THOMAS NELSON AND SONS LTD
Nelson House Mayfield Road
Walton-on-Thames Surrey KT12 5PL

P O Box 18123 Nairobi Kenya

116-D JTC Factory Building
Lorong 3 Geyland Square Singapore 1438

THOMAS NELSON AUSTRALIA PTY LTD
19–39 Jeffcott Street West Melbourne Victoria 3003

NELSON CANADA LTD
81 Curlew Drive Don Mills Ontario M3A 2R1

THOMAS NELSON (HONG KONG) LTD
Watson Estate Block A 13 Floor
Watson Road Causeway Bay Hong Kong

THOMAS NELSON (NIGERIA) LTD
8 Ilupeja Bypass PMB 21303 Ikeja Lagos

First published 1981
© J. Stephen and R. A. Pietrowski 1981

ISBN 0 17 771102 7

NCN 5812 42 0

Printed and bound in Hong Kong

Contents

Preface — vii

1 Introduction — 1

2 The sub-unit toxins — 9

Diphtheria toxin — 9
Pseudomonas aeruginosa toxins — 15
Cholera toxin — 16
Enterotoxins of *Escherichia coli* — 25
Neurotoxins: tetanus and botulinum toxins — 26
Colicins E3 and E2 — 33
Similar proteins of non-bacterial origin — 34
Summary — 35
References — 35

3 Membrane-damaging toxins; primary event defined — 36

Phospholipase activity — 37
Other phospholipases — 45
Thiol-activated cytolysins — 46
Toxins with a surfactant mechanism — 49
References — 49

4 Membrane-damaging toxins; primary event not known — 50

Staphylococcal toxins — 50
Streptococcal toxins — 57
Other membrane-damaging toxins — 58
Summary of Chapters 3 and 4 — 58
References — 58

5 Toxins of known importance in the genesis of specific lesions; mode of action not known — 59

Anthrax toxin — 59
Enterotoxins — 63
Clostridial toxins — 69
Streptococcal erythrogenic toxins — 75
Summary — 76
References — 77

Contents

6 Cell-associated toxins   **78**

Endotoxins   78
Toxins of *Yersinia pestis*   93
Summary   97
References   98

Glossary   **99**

Index   **102**

Preface

This book provides more than a lucid and up to date account of the molecular biology of bacterial toxins with commendable attention to distinguishing between what is known and what is speculation. In particular, and this should appeal to young students, it paints the picture of disease and its prevention in an interesting manner, before describing the nature and relevance of appropriate toxins. Also, better than in any other book I know, toxins are related to other determinants of pathogenicity which are often of equal importance in the disease process.

Harry Smith
Birmingham 1980

1 Introduction

Some 250 bacterial genera are listed in Bergey's *Manual of Determinative Bacteriology*, of which only approximately ten per cent include species which are pathogenic to man or animals. Not every species within a genus is pathogenic and not every strain of each pathogen is virulent, so the fraction of the total microbial biomass capable of causing disease must be very small. The basic metabolism of pathogens and non-pathogens is the same, so it follows that pathogens must possess highly specialized attributes which enable them to cause disease.

A pathogen must be able to enter the body, lodge in some primary site (and in some cases stay there), multiply in the changing pathophysiological conditions it induces, and out-compete existing commensals in the process. Some pathogens may spread to, or invade, other tissues. While this is happening the host is mounting non-specific (phagocytic cells and microbicidal body fluids) and specific (the immune system of antibodies and cells) host defence mechanisms, both of which must be overcome or evaded for the pathogen to be successful.

Ultimately, biochemical lesions with or without accompanying structural tissue damage occur which lead to overt disease and sometimes death. There are two principal mechanisms for causing damage. One involves the activation by microbial substances (which are often non-toxic by themselves) of components of the immune system, which does not always operate in a protective sense to the advantage of the host; this is known as hypersensitivity or immunopathological damage and is not dealt with in this book. The other mechanism involves the production of toxic substances which interact directly with appropriate targets; it is with this narrow aspect of the complex but fascinating subject of pathogenicity that this book is concerned.

The roots of our subject go back to the last quarter of the 19th century, a period which has understandably been called the golden age of microbiology. During this era, dominated by Pasteur in France, Koch in Germany and their illustrious colleagues, the causative organisms of many infectious diseases were isolated. From such beginnings the science of general microbiology emerged, but for years microbiologists were mainly concerned with that relatively small proportion of the incredibly diverse microbial world which affects the health of man and his domestic animals.

The two main goals sought by the early workers were means of immunizing susceptible hosts against disease and the discovery of toxins elaborated by pathogens and responsible for the production of disease. Pasteur, in the early 1880s exploited the use of attenuated organisms in protecting animals and man against fowl cholera, anthrax, and rabies. This use of live vaccines was possible because some organisms, when grown in laboratory media or in alternative hosts, become sufficiently avirulent to be injected live into susceptible species and thereby stimulate a protective immune response without causing overt disease. This approach was somewhat similar to that developed some 80 years previously by Jenner, who showed that inoculation of humans with cowpox conferred immunity against smallpox. We now know in retrospect what Jenner could not have known, that this is an example of generating immunity against a virulent virus by injecting another closely related but distinguishable avirulent virus. About the same time as Pasteur's work, Salmon and Smith in America demonstrated that heat-killed cultures of *Salmonella choleraesuis* protected pigeons against a lethal challenge dose of live organisms, thus showing that acquired immunity results from exposure to some constituent of the pathogen which could be produced in laboratory culture, as well as in the living tissues and fluids of animals.

In none of these examples was the mechanism responsible for the induction of acquired immunity understood. Pasteur's work on chicken cholera stemmed from a chance observation that cultures of the causative organism (*Pasteurella multocida*), which had been left to stand on the bench during a vacation, would no longer kill chickens. Moreover, chickens which had received the old cultures were not killed by injection of fresh cultures.

The development of antitoxin therapy, followed some 30 years later by prophylactic immunization with stable toxoids, was much less empirical. Advances stemmed from the observations of Loeffler, Roux and Yersin, Behring and Kitasato on the aetiology of diphtheria and tetanus, and of Ermengen on botulism. These diseases were demonstrably caused by powerful toxins which could be produced *in vitro* and, when introduced into experimental animals, reproduced the main features of the disease caused by live organisms.

By 1892, Behring had discovered antitoxins. In his search for antibacterial substances, he injected tetanus-infected animals with iodoform. This spared the animals but did not kill the organisms. He reasoned that the effect, therefore, must be on the toxin. Transfer of serum from animals so treated to fresh animals rendered the recipients resistant to the effects of toxin and led to the discovery of antitoxins, later recognized as proteins belonging to the immunoglobulin class of serum proteins.

The impact of these discoveries was enormous and stimulated much toxin-orientated research during the next 25 years. Serum therapy for diphtheria and tetanus was successfully developed using mainly horses for large scale production of antitoxin. Such success prompted further searches for similar substances to explain the principal features of other bacterial infections, and against which antitoxins could be generated for therapeutic use. For example, the great Koch, after his classic elucidation of the aetiology of tuberculosis, devoted considerable effort spanning some 15 years in attempts to isolate an antitubercular agent from *Mycobacterium tuberculosis*. Tuberculin, the product of this effort, proved to have neither therapeutic nor prophylactic efficacy, but only diagnostic value. There were many other fruitless searches.

For the next 25 years progress in bacterial toxinology was less dramatic. As a result of experience gained during World War I in treating soldiers whose wounds became infected with anaerobic bacteria (in particular with clostridial species) gas gangrene was added to the small number of diseases in which a toxin played a significant if not overriding role. Another development was the production in the 1920s by Glenny in Britain and Ramon in France of toxoids which are stable, chemically detoxified toxins safe for use in human prophylaxis. Recipients were thus actively immunized in that they produced their own antitoxins which would neutralize native toxins, as opposed to passively immunized, when they received antitoxin pre-formed in another species.

During this period, in which medical microbiology underwent descriptive and diagnostic consolidation, other research areas were opened up. At first these were

2

peripheral to the study of toxins and antitoxins but developed rapidly into the separate though inter-related disciplines of serology, immunology, and immunochemistry. Chemotherapy also originated from this period, the result of the pursuit by Ehrlich of another kind of specificity which resided in his concept of 'magic bullets'.

The decade from the late 1920s to the late 1930s saw some new developments in the field of bacterial toxins. Several species of clostridia, important in veterinary as well as human disease, were shown to produce a range of soluble antigens, some of which were toxic to experimental animals, and successful vaccines were developed.

Serological analysis of toxic culture filtrates was also developed for the classification of some clostridia. This led to the recognition of additional extracellular antigens, some of which were of potential relevance in the establishment and/or spread of infection. It is important to point out that many bacterial toxins (and other soluble antigens) were first recognized either by their biological activity or as serological entities. In many cases they were arbitrarily assigned a letter of the Greek alphabet. Thus we have α-toxins of *Clostridium perfringens*, *Clostridium novyi*, and staphylococci which are completely unrelated to each other in any way other than that they are designated alpha. Even more confusing is the fact that some toxins bearing different Greek symbols were subsequently shown to be serologically and/or biochemically related.

The onset of World War II stimulated further research into toxigenic anaerobes, particularly those belonging to the gas gangrene group of clostridia. Analysis of this disease was and still is complicated. Gas gangrene is frequently caused by a range of anaerobes (including *C. perfringens, C. novyi, C. septicum*) either alone or in combination. Moreover, *C. perfringens*, the most studied organism in this group, is one of the most prolific producers of toxins and other extracellular antigens of potential significance in pathogenicity among known bacteria. Despite these complexities, considerable attention was focused on the alpha toxin of *C. perfringens* with respect to development of a prophylactic toxoid because it was thought to be the most important of the several factors produced by allegedly the most important of the bacterial species concerned with gas gangrene. This toxin became the first for which a biochemical mode of action was recognized when, in 1941, Macfarlane and Knight showed it to be a phospholipase C enzyme (lecithinase in older literature) which split phosphoryl choline from the cell membrane component, phosphatidyl choline, in the presence of Ca^{2+} ions. However, its role in gas gangrene infections was not unequivocally established. Even more intriguing was the observation that not every bacterial species which produced phospholipase C was necessarily pathogenic, nor were all such enzymes equally toxic.

In the early 1950s microbial pathogenicity in general, and bacterial toxins in particular, again became productive areas of research. Smith and Keppie and their numerous colleagues at the Microbiological Research Establishment, Porton, England, launched a series of studies on pathogenic bacteria and their products derived from *in vivo* sources. The prevailing climate was the threat of biological warfare and how to combat it. One organism with military potential was *Bacillus anthracis*, an aerobic spore-forming organism which could, if disseminated, survive in the environment. It infects man (albeit poorly) as well as animals, for which it is a natural pathogen. But, no-one then knew anything about the lethal mechanisms of this pathogen. In 1955, the Porton group demonstrated the existence of a hitherto undiscovered toxin elaborated by *B. anthracis*. The discovery of anthrax toxin was in many ways a modern classic. First, it resulted in the elucidation of the principal bacterial determinant of fatal anthrax infections, something which had eluded discovery for many years. Second, it gave a kiss of life to a subject which was then almost moribund. It also defused the military potential of this pathogen.

The mid-, and immediately post-war years had seen the development of our knowledge and understanding of some gas gangrene toxins to a point where bacterial toxinology had been brought within the framework of prevailing biochemical concepts. However, at this point the momentum of phospolipase (lecithinase) work had waned, and Pappenheimer's ingenious idea that diphtheria toxin interfered with aspects of energy metabolism was displaced. In 1959 Strauss and Hendee set future investigators on the right trail by observing that diphtheria toxin in fact inhibited protein synthesis. Another significant observation was made in 1953 by De and his collaborators. They injected cell-free filtrates of *Vibrio cholerae* into the lumen of the rabbit ileum and demonstrated the accumulation of fluid. The active factor was a heat-labile protein fittingly described as an enterotoxin. However, it was some 17 years after De's original observation before the enterotoxin bandwagon really started to roll with its present momentum.

During the 1960s tremendous strides were made in our understanding of the mode of action of diphtheria toxin. Strauss and Hendee demonstrated the inhibition of protein synthesis in tissue culture cells by diphtheria toxin, and Collier, Honjo, Gill, Pappenheimer and their colleagues showed that the toxic protein consists of two fragments, one of which is enzymically active in splitting NAD^+ and transferring one of the cleavage products to, and thereby inactivating, a key enzyme involved in protein synthesis. The other fragment somehow facilitates the passage of the enzymic fragment across the normally impassable cell membrane.

Such brilliant studies brought to a molecular conclusion (some 80 years after the discovery of the toxin) work on certain aspects, probably the most important aspects, of the disease diphtheria which, because of enlightened immunization programmes, had already become a clinical rarity. But, just as important, these observations brought bacterial toxinology into the realms of protein sub-unit biochemistry and protein-membrane interactions, areas which are currently being rapidly developed and which provide a conceptual framework within which increasing numbers of other systems have been or may yet be interpreted.

The 1970s were a period of intense activity during which enterotoxins were examined in great detail. The initial surge came from the need to develop more effective vaccines to control outbreaks of cholera in areas where it is still endemic or in areas where natural disasters or the ravages of war create conditions conducive to the spread of the disease. Attention was focused on the enterotoxin discovered by De in 1953, and a massive programme was launched which resulted in our knowing more about the molecular pathology of cholera than any other infectious disease. Other enterobacteria also cause diarrhoea, probably by virtue of their ability to produce enterotoxins which in some cases are functionally (maybe structurally) similar to that produced by *V. cholerae*.

In retrospect, the discovery of toxins relevant in disease was easiest in those cases in which the toxin was a single extracellular protein, the principal determinant of disease production, and *killed* test animals irrespective of the route of injection. This explains why diphtheria, tetanus and botulinum toxins were discovered early on and also why so little success was achieved for years after, despite intensive searches for other toxins. Later work showed the importance of using the right test animal (or other appropriate system), and the right route and site of injection in searching for the biochemical determinants of cell and tissue damage. As will be exemplified later in this book, some problems in pathogenicity which possibly involve toxins remain unsolved because of the phenotypic plasticity and multifactorial nature of the virulence of the organisms concerned.

The current revival of interest in bacterial toxins also reflects the rapid expansion in knowledge of membrane structure. By the use of highly purified phospholipases of known specificity to modify membrane phospholipids, valuable information has been gained with respect to the asymmetric distribution of lipids between the outer and inner leaflets of the membrane. Such studies require enzymes of very high purity, otherwise it becomes impossible to interpret the observed effects on the treated membrane as primary effects of the enzyme, or of some active contaminant. As a result our knowledge about the production, purification, biochemical and physicochemical properties of phospholipases—which include bacterial toxins—has increased dramatically over recent years.

Some toxins are known, and others undoubtedly will yet be shown, to interact with specific receptors on susceptible cell membranes as a prelude to intracytoplasmic uptake or initiation of their toxic responses. Other toxins actually damage cell membranes themselves. Here we will briefly summarize those properties of membranes which are relevant in the context of the site and mode of toxin action (see Fig. 1).

The modern view of the molecular arrangements which give rise to the trilamellar appearance of cell membranes in the electron microscope is of a bimolecular leaflet comprising lipids and proteins; the asymmetric distribution of both lipids and proteins between the outer and inner layers is well established and the ratio of total lipid to protein varies enormously between cell types and also between organelles. Some proteins exist in only one half of the bilayer; others exist as transmembrane proteins having one or more polypeptide sub-units and are in contact with both the inside and outside of the cell. The inner half of the membrane is linked to contractile elements—filaments and microtubules—which comprise the cytoskeletal system

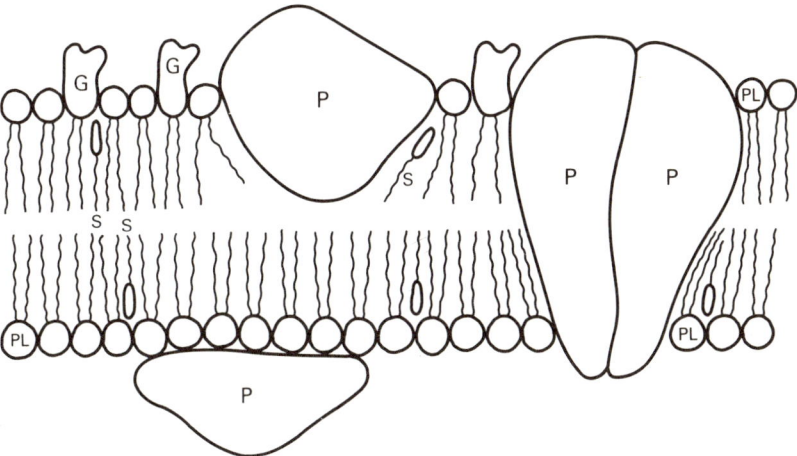

Figure 1 Schematic representation of cell membrane P: protein; PL: phospholipid; G: ganglioside; S: sterol.

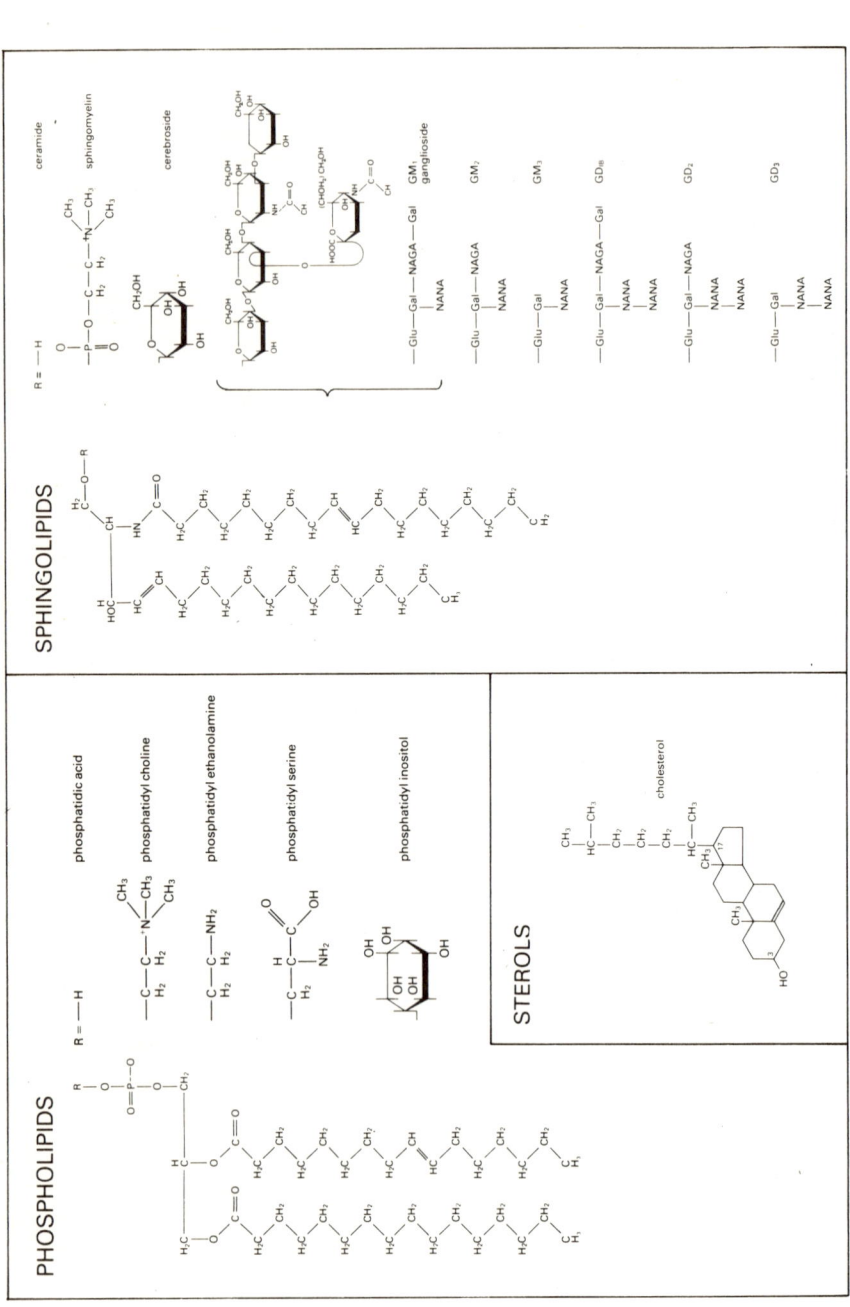

Figure 2 Membrane constituents

6

responsible for endocytotic phenomena and cell motility. Lateral diffusion of membrane constituents can occur but, in contrast, vertical passive movement across membranes occurs much less frequently, being mainly restricted to certain compounds of low molecular weight or of relatively high hydrophobicity. However, as we shall see, some toxins possess a special mechanism for reaching their intracytoplasmic target sites.

The most important classes of lipids from our point of view are phospholipids, sphingolipids, glycolipids, cerebrosides, gangliosides and sterols, whose structures and formal derivation are shown in Fig. 2.

It is not possible to proceed without defining the term toxin, a task which is more difficult than one might think. In 1954, Oakley suggested that the term had outlived its usefulness and should be replaced by 'soluble bacterial antigen', a suggestion which, despite the eminence of its author, never caught on. The term has survived another 25 years without its being defined in a manner which is accurate and which commands universal approval; it looks like remaining for another 25 years. The most eloquent of recent attempts was that of Bonventre (1970) who defined toxins as a 'special class' of poisons which differ from, for example, cyanide or mercury by virtue of their microbial origin, protein structure, high molecular weight, and antigenicity. In the context of disease this view is both too embracing, because it includes proteins of doubtful significance in disease, and too restrictive, because it excludes non-protein toxic complexes such as endotoxin. He further proposed that toxins should be classified either according to their function in the organism from which they are derived, their mode of action in the host, or their molecular structure. The first criterion is difficult to apply except perhaps for toxins which are known structural entities in the bacterial cell and which therefore must have some important structural or metabolic significance. The second is attractive but is also difficult because the fact that one can ascribe a specific enzymic action to one toxin does not mean that all enzymes of the same biochemical specificity are toxic. Moreover, the modes of action of many toxins are unknown. The third suggestion is difficult when one attempts to embrace within a nomenclatural system toxins which are synthesized as inactive precursors which undergo activation, and others which are complex mixtures of different components.

Another suggestion is that toxin must include all naturally occurring substances (of plant, animal, bacterial or whatever origin) which when introduced into a foreign host are adverse to the well-being or life of the victim. This, too, is problematical since some substances—toxins within the scope of this definition—are used in some contexts as therapeutic agents. It seems pointless to attempt an all-embracing definition covering all naturally occurring toxic products or even all microbial toxins. The obvious differences between bacterial and fungal toxins warrant the continued use of the appropriate prefix. For example, bacterial toxins are usually of high molecular weight and hence antigenic, whereas fungal toxins tend to be low molecular weight and not antigenic. We shall side-step the semantic issue and follow a more pragmatic line, but this, too, has its problems.

Difficulties arise from attempting to define a term embracing substances (aggressins) which help to establish an infective focus as well as those whose action is uniquely or largely responsible for the disease syndrome. These problems are compounded when one is faced with the decision of including or excluding a variety of substances known to be produced by bacteria *in vitro*—and whose properties on *a priori* grounds make them potentially significant as determinants of disease—but whose production or role in the establishment of an infection *in vivo* has not yet been

7

established. The thiol-activated cytolysins produced by several bacterial species are a classic example; there are others.

Primary consideration will be given, therefore, to those substances which are produced under ecologically significant conditions and cause damage to cells, tissues or the whole animal, thereby contributing to, or being the major cause of, disease. The discussions of topics which are controversial or which have not yet been clarified will be guided by criteria set out in 1955 by van Heyningen, which are still helpful in deciding whether or not a toxin plays a role in disease. Does the organism produce the toxin *in vivo*? Is there a correlation between virulence and toxigenicity? Is it possible to demonstrate sterile lesions in the infected animal, particularly at a site distant from the foci of bacterial multiplication? Does injection of sterile toxin preparations reproduce signs that mimic the disease? Can the course of the disease be altered by therapeutic administration of antitoxin or can the initiation of the disease be prevented by prophylactic use of antitoxin which may be passively administered or actively induced? These are idealized criteria, the application and limitations of which will be discussed in relation to specific examples.

References

AJL, S. J., KADIS, S., MONTI, T. C., & WEINBAUM, J. Eds. (1970, 1971). *Microbial Toxins.* Vols I–V. Academic Press.

BONVENTRE, P. F. (1970). 'Nomenclature of microbial toxins: problems and recommendations.' In: *Microbial Toxins,* Vol. I. p. 29 Edited by S. J. Ajl, S. Kadis and T. C. Montie. Academic Press.

LECHEVALIER, H. A. & SOLOTOROVSKY, M. (1965). *Three centuries of microbiology.* McGraw Hill, New York.

MIMS, C. A. (1976). *The pathogenesis of infectious disease.* Academic Press, London.

Mechanisms of microbial pathogenicity. (1955). Vth Symposium of the Society of General Microbiology. Edited by J. W. Howie and A. J. O'Hea (Articles by A. A. Miles, W. E. van Heyningen, M. G. Macfarlane are relevant; others are out of date.)

2 The sub-unit toxins

This chapter is devoted principally to a small, heterogeneous group of bacterial toxins whose unifying feature is a special relationship between toxin structure and function. With one, perhaps two exceptions, the toxins discussed consist of two distinct non-identical protein moieties. Where the molecular mode of action of these toxins has been elucidated, it seems that one protein moiety binds the toxin to susceptible cells and in some way facilitates the entry of the second protein moiety into the cytoplasm where it exerts its lethal action.

We shall consider in detail two toxins, diphtheria and cholera toxin, whose structural and functional properties are well understood and then outline briefly the properties of other toxins where they are known to differ from, or have not as yet been shown to conform with, the general features of diphtheria and cholera toxin.

Diphtheria toxin

Although the causative organism of diphtheria, *Corynebacterium diphtheriae*, can normally be isolated only from the characteristic membranous* lesion found in the throat, autopsy of fatal cases reveals widespread necrotic and haemorrhagic lesions in many organs of the body. These lesions were first shown in 1888 to be caused by a potent, extracellular, heat-labile toxin produced by bacteria in the nasopharynx and transported throughout the body by the bloodstream. The finding in 1890 that antibodies raised against this toxin protect against the disease itself, and the later discovery that treatment of diphtheria toxin with dilute formalin renders the molecule non-toxic without impairing its serological and immunogenic properties, led to a programme of mass-immunization and the virtual eradication of what was formerly a major cause of death, especially among children. However, it is only in the last two decades that we have begun to understand the pathogenesis of the disease at the molecular level.

The molecule is highly toxic for many animal species including man, rabbits, guinea pigs, and some birds; as little as 50–100 ng toxin per kg body weight is lethal. In general the toxin is relatively non-selective in its tissue specificity. Rats, mice, and cell lines derived from these animals are very resistant to the toxin.

Toxin synthesis; lysogeny Diphtheria toxin is produced only by strains of *C. diphtheriae* infected with lysogenic bacteriophages which carry within their genome the *tox* gene. Non-toxigenic strains of *C. diphtheriae* can be made toxigenic by infection with any one of several morphologically and serologically distinct classes of corynephages carrying the *tox* gene; certain related species such as *Corynebacterium ovis* can also be made toxigenic. Furthermore, infection with corynephages having a mutation in the *tox* gene leads to synthesis of mutant toxin molecules which lack, or possess diminished, toxicity but which react serologically

* Gr., *diphthera* = membrane.

9

with antitoxin and are thus called cross-reacting materials (CRMs). This indicates that the product of the *tox* gene is diphtheria toxin itself and not just a molecule required to 'turn on' a structural gene carried by the bacterial host. Thus, we are drawn to the fascinating conclusion that the major virulence factor of *C. diphtheriae* is coded for not by the bacterium but by an infecting virus. However, the bacterium is responsible for the regulation of the expression of this gene and thus different strains of *C. diphtheriae* infected with the same phage vary greatly in their yield of toxin under optimal conditions, a process intimately related to intracellular iron content. In most strains, little or no toxin is synthesized *in vitro* until the late stages of growth when the iron content of the medium is virtually exhausted and the intracellular iron content begins to decrease. Under these conditions approximately 35 per cent of the total protein synthesized by the avirulent Park Williams 8 strain of *C. diphtheriae* is toxin.

The molecular basis for this regulation is now beginning to be understood. If DNA from a converting corynephage such as *β-tox⁺* is added to *Escherichia coli* cell-free protein synthesizing systems, toxin production is unaffected by iron concentration. However, the addition of even very small amounts of a cell-free extract from a non-toxigenic strain of *C. diphtheriae* inhibits *tox* gene expression in the *E. coli* system. The factor responsible has been partly purified and shown to be an iron-containing protein which, in the presence of iron, binds to DNA. Thus, corynebacterial cells apparently contain a *tox* gene repressor which requires iron as a co-repressor. This may not be the only role of this protein in the bacterium because it is also present in non-toxigenic strains.

It is interesting to speculate about the origin of the *tox* gene, since its product, although carried by corynephages, plays no part in the replication and assembly of these viruses and is therefore apparently superfluous to the particles' requirements. However, the virtual disappearance of toxigenic strains of *C. diphtheriae* as commensals in the nasopharynx since the commencement of mass immunization suggests that toxin production is essential for survival of the bacterium and therefore of the virus.

According to one suggestion the *tox* gene arose by modification of an existing phage gene. Since any modification would result in the loss of the original gene product, this presupposes that the original gene was itself non-essential for replication and assembly, a view which conflicts with our concept of the simplicity of bacteriophages. This apparent drawback can be circumvented by the model for molecular evolution proposed by Hartley. This supposes that because most mutations in a single gene will be disadvantageous, gene duplication must first occur to allow mutations to accumulate in one copy without the essential genetic complement being diminished. In support of this hypothesis, limited evidence suggests that one corynephage virion protein does in fact bear similarities to diphtheria toxin.

A further suggestion is that the *tox* gene may have been acquired from some other bacterial source. The position of *tox* near one end of the phage genome supports such a suggestion, as does the observation that the *tox* gene is carried by a variety of morphologically and serologically unrelated corynephages. It is unlikely that the same gene modification has taken place in all the different kinds of phages; it is more likely that the gene has been distributed between the phages by recombination during multiple infection.

This relationship between toxigenicity and lysogeny is not confined to *C. diphtheriae*. Other toxins known to be coded for by lysogenic phages include botulinum toxin types C and D, *Clostridium novyi* α-toxin, and streptococcal erythrogenic toxin. Another group of toxins coded for by transmissable plasmids includes *E. coli* heat-labile and heat-stable enterotoxins, and staphylococcal exfoliatin serotype ii.

Cytotoxic activity Studies of the mode of action of diphtheria toxin have been advanced greatly by the use of animal cells in culture, which are more convenient to work with, are extremely sensitive to the toxin, and exhibit the same relative susceptibility to the toxin as the animals from which they are derived.

In 1959, Strauss and Hendee showed that, after a latent period of 1–1.5 h, protein synthesis in HeLa cells is drastically inhibited by diphtheria toxin. Others showed that, in cell-free extracts, inhibition of protein synthesis is dependent upon the presence of NAD$^+$ and is effected by inactivation of a protein essential for eukaryotic protein synthesis, elongation factor 2 (EF2). By incubating EF2 with diphtheria toxin and NAD$^+$ radioactively labelled in different parts of the molecule, it was subsequently shown that the toxin inhibits protein synthesis by catalysing the transfer of the ADP-ribose moiety from NAD$^+$ to a single amino acid residue of EF2, which is thus inactivated (Fig. 3). Diphtheria toxin is an enzyme: one molecule inside a cell inactivates many molecules of EF2, and will kill a susceptible cell within 24 h.

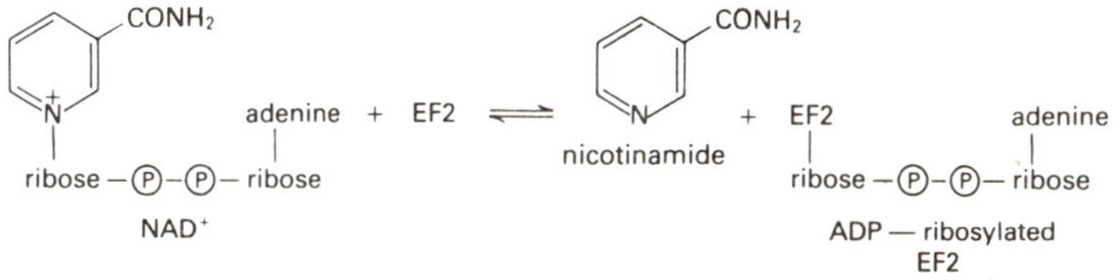

Figure 3 Mechanism of inactivation of elongation factor 2 (EF2) by diphtheria toxin

Is ADP-ribosylation of EF2 the lethal event *in vivo*? Bonventre and Imhoff in 1966 showed a marked inhibition of protein synthetic capacity in cardiac and pancreatic tissues of guinea pigs injected with lethal doses of diphtheria toxin. This strongly suggested that death *in vivo* is the result of inhibition of protein synthesis, but is ADP-ribosylation of EF2 the cause of this inhibition? Bonventre reasoned that because ADP-ribosylation is a catalytic reaction and therefore reversible, incubation of untreated ribosomes with soluble extracts of intoxicated tissue in the presence of excess nicotinamide should lead to reactivation of the ADP-ribosylated target protein and the restoration of protein synthetic activity. Bowman and Bonventre subsequently demonstrated that this occurred and concluded that death *in vivo* from diphtheria toxin stems from inhibition of protein synthesis, primarily in heart tissue, caused by ADP-ribosylation of a soluble protein, in all probability EF2.

As EF2 is a cytoplasmic protein, it is obvious that the site of action of diphtheria toxin is intracellular. Thus, the toxin must traverse the cell membrance to expose its catalytic site to, or enter the cytoplasm before the inhibition of protein synthesis.

11

Structure-function relationships The first evidence suggesting a relationship between structure and function in the diphtheria toxin molecule came from work, primarily by Collier and his associates, in the late 1960s. They found that preparations of diphtheria toxin often contain a low molecular weight protein which is far more active than the whole toxin in inhibiting protein synthesis in cell-free systems. Further investigation showed that the whole toxin is a pro-enzyme with all the ADP-ribosylating activity residing in a non-toxic proteolytic fragment of approximate molecular weight 22 000 daltons.

Further work led to the presently accepted concept of the structure of diphtheria toxin. It has a molecular weight of 62–63 000 daltons and is synthesized as a single polypeptide containing two disulphide bonds. The region between the disulphide bond nearest the NH_2-terminus of the protein contains three arginine residues which are very susceptible to proteolytic cleavage by trypsin. Such cleavage or 'nicking' yields two polypeptide fragments held together by a single disulphide bond and weak non-covalent interactions. Treatment of the 'nicked' toxin with thiol agents such as 2-mercaptoethanol or dithiothreitol yields, under dissociating conditions, two polypeptide fragments, designated A and B (Fig. 4).

The A fragment has a molecular weight of approximately 22 000 daltons and is exceedingly stable, withstanding short periods of boiling and extremes of pH without appreciable loss of activity. The fragment carries all the ADP-ribosylating activity of the toxin and is a potent inhibitor of protein synthesis in eukaryotic cell-free systems. However, it has less than 0.01 per cent of the toxicity of intact toxin for whole cells, indicating that the rest of the toxin molecule serves a role in effecting the transport of fragment A from the surrounding medium into the cell cytoplasm where it exerts its toxic activity. Antibodies prepared against A fragment do not neutralize whole toxin, which suggests that antigenic sites on the A fragment are masked by the B fragment in the whole toxin.

Fragment B has a molecular weight of approximately 40 000 daltons and inhibits protein synthesis in neither whole cells nor cell-free extracts. In contrast to A, it is very unstable in normal aqueous buffers and until recently was reported to be soluble only in the presence of strong dissociating agents such as urea, guanidine, or the detergent sodium dodecylsulphate (SDS). For this reason, knowledge of the structure and properties of the B fragment was initially restricted to that gleaned from the study of defective toxins such as CRM_{197} which has a functional B fragment but defective A fragment. This competitively inhibits the toxic effect of whole toxin for cells in culture, suggesting that susceptible cells possess specific receptors to which diphtheria toxin binds *via* the B fragment. Recently, soluble stable B fragment has been prepared without recourse to denaturants, and competition experiments have confirmed that the B fragment alone is responsible for the binding of diphtheria toxin to specific receptors and, in addition, active toxin has been resynthesized from purified dissociated fragments.

Studies of the kinetics of toxin binding reveal that each susceptible HeLa cell possesses approximately 4000 specific receptors. This figure is low in comparison with the number of receptors for, say, cholera toxin. Mouse and rat cells are resistant to diphtheria toxin because they lack specific receptors. The nature of the toxin receptor is as yet unknown. However, by treating susceptible cells with toxin, solubilizing the cells and then immunoprecipitating the toxin-receptor complex, Hart has shown that diphtheria toxin binds specifically to a protein of molecular weight 120–170 000 daltons which is not present on the surface of resistant mouse L cells.

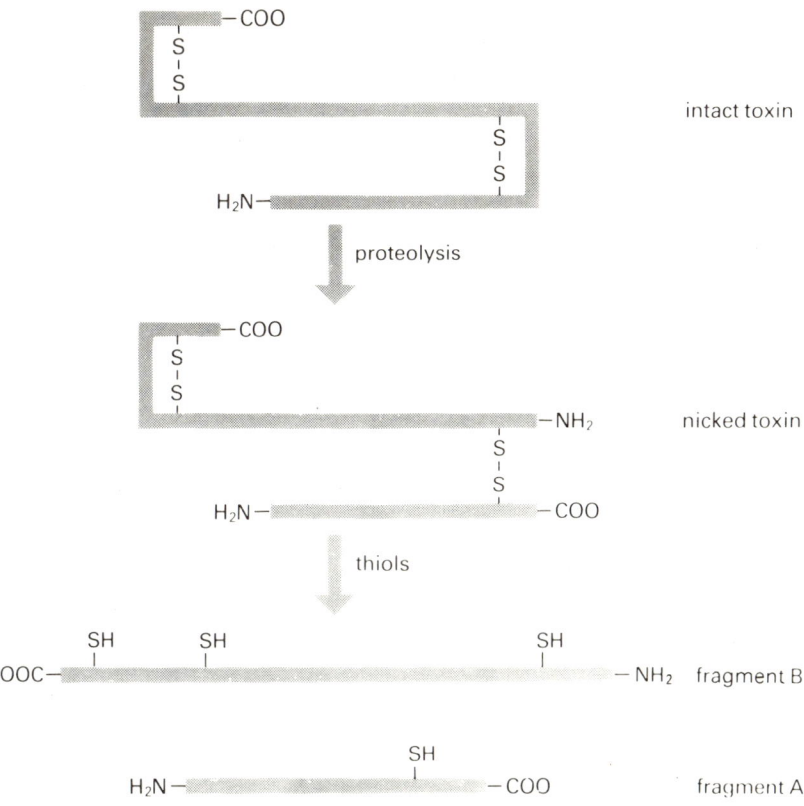

Figure 4 The structure of diphtheria toxin. The toxin is synthesized as a single poly-peptide but is easily cleaved, or 'nicked', by proteases into two fragments, designated A and B, held together by a readily reducible disulphide bond.

Mechanism of entry About the only thing we can say with certainty about the mechanism by which diphtheria toxin enters susceptible cells is that it proceeds from an initial interaction between specific receptors on the cell surface and the B fragment. Beyond this, information is negative and ideas conjectural. Binding is not inhibited by trypsin or pronase, hence the receptor is not an easily accessible surface protein; nor is it inhibited by neuraminidase or hyaluronidase, suggesting that binding is not to the sialic or hyaluronic acid residues of, for example, membrane glycoproteins.

One interesting observation is that entry and subsequent killing of cells by diphtheria toxin can be inhibited by low concentrations of ammonium salts, a phenomenon peculiar to diphtheria toxin uptake as far as is known. However, entry is known to be very sensitive to pH, and it has been suggested that the ammonium ions may merely be bringing about pH changes at the cell surface. Inhibitors of energy metabolism (and hence endocytosis) do not inhibit entry of diphtheria toxin, arguing against endocytosis as the predominant entry mechanism.

13

Boquet and Pappenheimer observed that the non-toxic CRM_{45}, a molecule having a functional A fragment but lacking the COOH-terminal 17 000 dalton amino acid sequence of the B fragment, is incapable of binding to susceptible cells. From this they suggested that this COOH-terminal portion of the fragment is responsible for binding to specific receptors. (This conclusion may not be fully justified as this portion of the B fragment may be required to maintain the necessary configuration for appropriate amino acid residues throughout the fragment to interact with the receptor.) Also, by observing the extent of binding of radioactively labelled detergent to CRM_{45} and intact toxin, Boquet and Pappenheimer estimated the ability of these proteins to interact hydrophobically with membranes. The two proteins bound equal amounts of detergent, from which it was deduced that there exists a hydrophobic domain in the 23 000 dalton amino acid sequence of B that is linked to the A fragment and capable of interacting with the cell membrane.

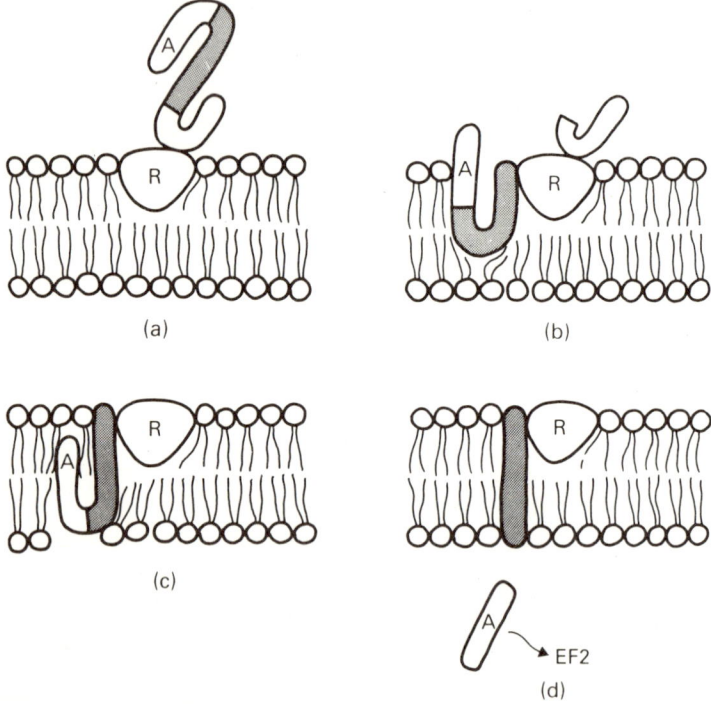

(a)

(b)

(c)

(d)

Figure 5 Proposed mechanism by which diphtheria toxin A fragment traverses the membrane of susceptible cells. An initial reversible interaction between specific receptors and groups located on the 17000 dalton COOH-terminal portion of the B fragment (a) is followed by an irreversible step which involves a conformational change in the toxin, possibly entailing the removal of the hydrophilic COOH-terminal polypeptide (b) and insertion into the membrane of the hydrophobic portion of the B fragment, which draws the A fragment through the lipid bilayer to the inner membrane surface (c). Within the membrane, proteases cleave the toxin into its constituent fragments, and thiol agents split the disulphide bond between the fragments and allow the release of A fragment into the cytoplasm, where it rapidly inhibits protein synthesis (d).

Based on this information, Boquet and Pappenheimer suggested a two-step entry mechanism for diphtheria toxin. An initial reversible interaction between specific receptors and groups located on the 17 000 dalton COOH-terminal portion of the B fragment is followed by an irreversible step which involves a conformational change in the toxin, possibly entailing the removal of the hydrophilic COOH-terminal polypeptide. The hydrophobic portion of the B fragment is then inserted into the membrane which presumably draws the A fragment through the lipid bilayer to the inner membrane surface. Within the membrane, proteases cleave the toxin into its constituent fragments and thiol enzymes split the disulphide bond between the fragments and allow the release of A fragment into the cytoplasm, where it rapidly inhibits protein synthesis (Fig. 5). This entry mechanism is speculative but compatible with our present knowledge of the structure and properties of the diphtheria toxin molecule.

Pseudomonas aeruginosa toxins

Pseudomonas aeruginosa is common in soil and water and can occasionally be isolated from the faeces of normal, healthy individuals. It is virtually harmless for healthy adults, but its ability to multiply in almost any moist environment, and its resistance to many antibiotics, have made the bacterium a major cause of hospital-acquired infection, particularly among patients with impaired host-defence mechanisms such as those with chronic illness, genetic immunodeficiencies, those under treatment with immunosuppressive drugs, or patients suffering from extensive burns. *P. aeruginosa* causes localized infections in the urinary tract, respiratory tract, burns, and wound infections. In severely debilitated patients these localized infections may develop into general septicaemia, with mortality in such cases approaching 100 per cent.

Exotoxin A The mechanisms of pathogenicity of *P. aeruginosa* are complicated and unclear because the organism elaborates several potentially toxic extracellular products, including a phospholipase, collagenase, lipase, haemolysin, and enterotoxin as well as lipopolysaccharide endotoxin. However, increasing evidence suggests that a protein toxin, similar to diphtheria toxin, may be an important virulence factor. It is the most toxic product of *P. aeruginosa* and is produced by over 90 per cent of clinically important isolates. The toxin is produced during infection and specific antibodies can be detected in persons recuperating from infection. Antitoxin in some cases protects against infection in animals. Finally, non-toxigenic strains of *P. aeruginosa* are reported to be less virulent in experimental infection.

In 1969, Liu isolated the heat-labile toxin, designated exotoxin A, from filtrates of *P. aeruginosa* cultures and showed that injection of this into mice produced symptoms similar to those observed in animals infected with live organisms. Further work showed that antiserum against exotoxin A could in some cases protect mice and dogs against the lethal effects of challenge with live bacteria.

Iglewski and Kabat discovered, in 1975, that exotoxin A was in many ways like diphtheria toxin. It inhibits protein synthesis by ADP-ribosylation of EF2, is synthesized predominantly during the decline phase of cell growth, and its production appears to be dependent upon the concentration of iron in the medium. Its molecular weight is 66–70 000 daltons, and it can be activated in cell-free systems by proteolysis, by denaturation and reduction with thiols, or by freezing and thawing. All the enzymic activity of the toxin resides in a proteolytically derived fragment of molecular weight approximately 26 000 daltons. Thus, while we do not yet know whether the toxin consists of two distinct sub-units analogous to the A and B subunits of diphtheria toxin, we do know that the polypeptide is composed of functionally distinct regions. Several important dissimilarities exist between exotoxin A and diphtheria toxin, however. The two toxins are antigenically distinct, showing no serological cross-reactivity. Unlike diphtheria A fragment, the enzymically active fragment of exotoxin A is heat-labile. The defective diphtheria toxin molecule CRM_{197}, does not compete with exotoxin A for binding sites on whole cells, indicating that the two toxins have different receptors. Moreover, cell lines derived from mice are more sensitive to exotoxin A than are HeLa cells. At present we know nothing of the location of the *tox* gene, the nature of the toxin receptor, or the mechanism of entry of the enzymically active fraction into the cytoplasm.

Exoenzyme S Iglewski has recently identified another extracellular product of pathogenic strains of *P. aeruginosa* possessing ADP-ribosylating activity, which she has designated exoenzyme S. The protein is antigenically distinct from exotoxin A and is comparatively heat stable. It does not ADP-ribosylate EF2 (or EF1) but does ribosylate several red blood cell proteins, suggesting that its substrate probably has nothing to do with protein synthesis. The role of exoenzyme S in infection is unknown.

Cholera toxin

Cholera is an acute diarrhoeal disease which has been endemic to India and the Ganges basin for centuries: epidemics have spread from there to other parts of the world with devastating effects. Seven world-wide pandemics have occurred since the beginning of the nineteenth century, the latest spreading from Indonesia in 1959 to a total of 41 countries in Asia, Africa, and Eastern Europe by the early 1970s.

Vibrio cholerae was identified as the causative agent as long ago as 1854 by Pacini, but many bacteriologists remained sceptical of his findings and of the later observations by Koch, because similar but harmless vibrios could be isolated from a wide variety of environments.

Man usually contracts cholera from water or food which has been contaminated by faeces of a cholera victim. The ingested bacteria multiply in the alimentary canal and after 2–5 days cause the sudden onset of nausea, vomiting, acute diarrhoea, and abdominal cramp. In severe cases, the loss of fluid from the gut—in the form of liquid faeces referred to very descriptively as 'rice-water stools'—may be as great as 20 litres per day, leading to extreme dehydration. Shock frequently intervenes and death may occur within a few hours. Without adequate therapy the mortality rate may be as high as 60 per cent, but can be reduced to less than 1 per cent by intravenous replacement of fluid and electrolyte losses. Regardless of severity, the symptoms of the disease rarely last for more than a few days and biopsy of the intestine of cholera victims reveals only hyperaemia and superficial inflammation. Unlike diarrhoeas due to shigellae, the mucosa remains intact and the organisms do not invade the epithelium.

The discovery of the toxin Koch's suggestion that the symptoms of cholera were caused by a potent exotoxin secreted by the organisms in the gut, was unaccepted until the work of De and his colleagues in the 1950s showed that injection of *V. cholerae* or sterile culture filtrates into ligated segments of rabbit ileal loops *in vivo* leads to rapid accumulation of fluid in the lumen and consequent distention of the loop. However, further developments were surprisingly slow until the purification of the toxin in 1969 by Finklestein and his colleagues enabled the pathogenesis of cholera to be investigated at the molecular level.

Mode of action Our first real understanding of the mode of action of cholera toxin came from the work of Field, who measured the potential difference across stripped segments of ileal mucosa using an Ussing chamber (Fig. 6). In 1968, Field and his co-workers reported that the addition of cyclic AMP to the basal surface of short-circuited segments of ileal mucosa rapidly caused an increase in the short-circuit current. The direction of chloride ion transport was reversed (as judged by changes in the specific activity of radioactive NaCl in the Ringer solution) such that there was active secretion of chloride from the mucosal surface. Absorption of sodium ions was also reduced. Such changes in ion balance could bring about a passive efflux of water from the mucosal surface of the tissue and hence cause diarrhoea. Field saw the potential significance of this and the following year he reported that,

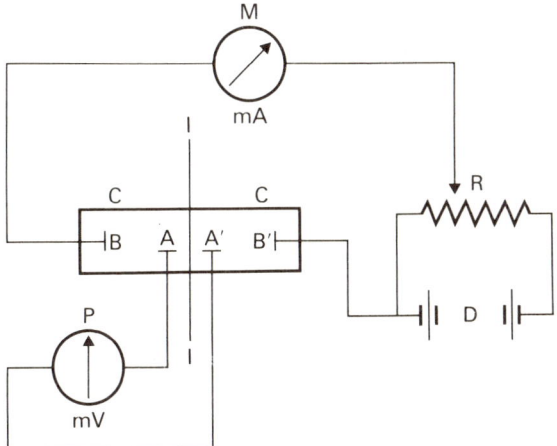

Figure 6 Ussing chamber. Viable tissue, when in contact on both sides with a physiological saline solution such as Ringer solution, maintains for many hours a potential difference between the inside and the outside, the inside of the cells being often more than 100 mV positive relative to the outside. The ileal mucosa (I) is placed as a membrane separating the Ringer solutions in chamber C. Two small electrodes (A and A') in the vicinity of the mucosa detect the potential difference across the tissue which is recorded by potentiometer (P). Another pair of electrodes (B and B') are attached to an external e.m.f. (D). By means of the rheostat (R) the voltage from D can be adjusted so that the potential difference across the tissue, as read on the potentiometer (P), is zero. This is equal to a total short-circuiting of the mucosal potential. The current passing through the mucosa at zero potential difference (the short-circuit current) is read on the milli-ammeter (M).

under the same conditions, sterile filtrates of cultures of *V. cholerae* mimicked exactly the effects of cyclic AMP and he suggested that the toxin acted *via* a mechanism related to cyclic AMP.

Later, using purified cholera toxin, Shafer and his colleagues demonstrated an increase in cyclic AMP in intoxicated tissue, and Sharp and Hynie subsequently found, in 1971, that cholera toxin stimulates adenylate cyclase activity in intestinal mucosa preparations. Thus, the physiological mechanism of cholera toxin activity was understood, superficially at least: the toxin caused diarrhoea by stimulating adenylate cyclase activity in the intestinal tract, thereby altering ion transport at the mucosal surface.

Cholera toxin mimics the various biological effects of cyclic AMP in every tissue so far examined. This has led to the development of several convenient *in vitro* assays for the toxin such as the induction of morphological changes (elongation) in cultured chinese hamster ovary (CHO) cells, and steroidogenesis in adrenal cortex cells.

Structure Finklestein and his colleagues first demonstrated that cholera toxin, or 'choleragen', is a protein having a molecular weight of approximately 84 000 daltons. Their toxin preparations were frequently contaminated with a smaller protein (molecular weight 56 000 daltons) which was non-toxic but serologically identical to cholera toxin. This was assumed to be a naturally occurring toxoid, or 'choleragenoid'. The existence of a non-toxic, serologically related protein of lower molecular weight suggested that cholera toxin possessed a sub-unit structure, perhaps similar to that of diphtheria toxin, which was by then under intensive study. This was confirmed by electrophoresis in the presence of SDS, which showed cholera toxin to consist of two protein moieties: one of molecular weight 28 000 daltons designated A, and the other 56 000 daltons (and apparently identical to choleragenoid) and designated B. More effective dissociating conditions revealed the 56 000 dalton moiety to be an aggregate of five smaller proteins (11 000 daltons) and that the 28 000 dalton moiety could be converted with thiols to two proteins of molecular weight 23 000 and 5000 daltons designated as A_1 and A_2 fragments respectively. Thus, like diphtheria toxin, cholera toxin is composed of two types of protein moiety, A and B. Unlike diphtheria toxin, however, the A and B sub-units are associated by non-covalent bonds. The A sub-unit is thought to be synthesized as a single polypeptide which undergoes subsequent proteolytic cleavage, in much the same way as diphtheria toxin, and for this reason the A_1 and A_2 polypeptides are referred to as protein *fragments*, whereas the A and B moieties of cholera toxin are called protein *sub-units*. Although each B sub-unit of cholera toxin contains an easily reducible disulphide bond, it is only accessible to chemical modification under extreme denaturing conditions, suggesting that the non-covalent internal protein-protein interactions maintaining the tertiary structure of the sub-unit are extremely strong.

The five B sub-units of cholera toxin form a very stable pentamer structure, so it is likely that the sub-unit—sub-unit interactions are all equal. The only way that such a stable pentameric structure can be achieved is by the formation of a closed ring with a central hole. The single A sub-unit is presumably located approximately on the axis of this ring, with fragment A_2 extending some distance into the central hole (Fig. 7). This model is supported by electron microscope evidence.

The A sub-unit is probably linked to the B region of the toxin by non-covalent association between the A_2 fragment and some of the B sub-units. The A_2 fragment

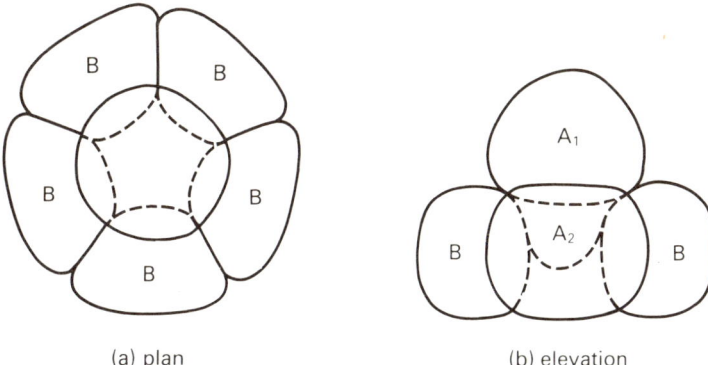

(a) plan   (b) elevation

Figure 7 The arrangement of the sub-units of cholera toxin. The five B sub-units form a ring structure (a) into which the A sub-unit partially inserts (b)

is thought not to be large enough to associate with all the B sub-units simultaneously. Chemical evidence that such a structure exists comes from the studies of Gill, who found that chemical cross-linking of the B pentamer was decreased in the presence of the A sub-unit. Presumably, the extension of A into the central hole of the B ring structure restricts cross-linking across this region. Furthermore, cross-linked oligomers, particularly trimers, of B sub-units run as very diffuse bands on polyacrylamide gel electrophoresis even in the presence of denaturing agents, suggesting that the sample comprises linear oligomers linked by tangential bonds and also of triangular structures containing cross-links that must have been formed across the centre of a hole-like region in the original pentamer. Obviously these oligomers would have different shapes and would therefore travel at different rates during electrophoresis.

Function of sub-units The B sub-units of cholera toxin, like the B fragment of diphtheria toxin, are non-toxic to cells: they possess no adenylate cyclase stimulating activity. They are responsible for the specific binding of cholera toxin to cells, since choleragenoid competes with whole toxin for binding sites on susceptible cells. The activity of cholera toxin is specifically and reversibly inhibited by low concentrations of the monosialoganglioside, GM_1 (see Fig. 2). The role of GM_1 as receptor for cholera toxin binding is strengthened by the observation that toxin-resistant cell lines, which lack GM_1 in the cell membrane, can be made sensitive to the toxin by the incorporation of GM_1 into the cell membrane.

The A sub-unit of cholera toxin is required for the stimulation of adenylate cyclase by cholera toxin. Avian erythrocytes have been used widely for *in vitro* studies of cholera toxin activity since these cells are easy to obtain in bulk, are easy to lyse and then fractionate into ghosts and cytoplasm, are metabolically simple and, most important, have a low basal rate of adenylate cyclase activity which can be increased manyfold by incubation with cholera toxin after lysis. In cell-free systems the A_1 fragment of the A sub-unit activates pigeon erythrocyte adenylate cyclase present in ghost membranes when NAD^+, nucleotide triphosphate (particularly GTP), and an unidentified cytosol protein are present. Under these conditions fragment A_1 exhibits ADP-ribosylating activity similar to that of the A fragment of diphtheria toxin.

Cassel and Pfeuffer in Germany, and Gill and Meren at Harvard, showed that in the pigeon erythrocyte system the target for ADP-ribosylation appears to be a protein of molecular weight 42–43 000 daltons. Ribosylation of this protein *always* occurs when adenylate cyclase is stimulated and *only* when it is stimulated, suggesting that activation is brought about by ADP-ribosylation of some component of the adenylate cyclase system. Support for this theory comes from the observation that, at maximum levels of ADP-ribosylation, approximately 1500 target proteins per pigeon erythocyte ghost are ADP-ribosylated; this is in good

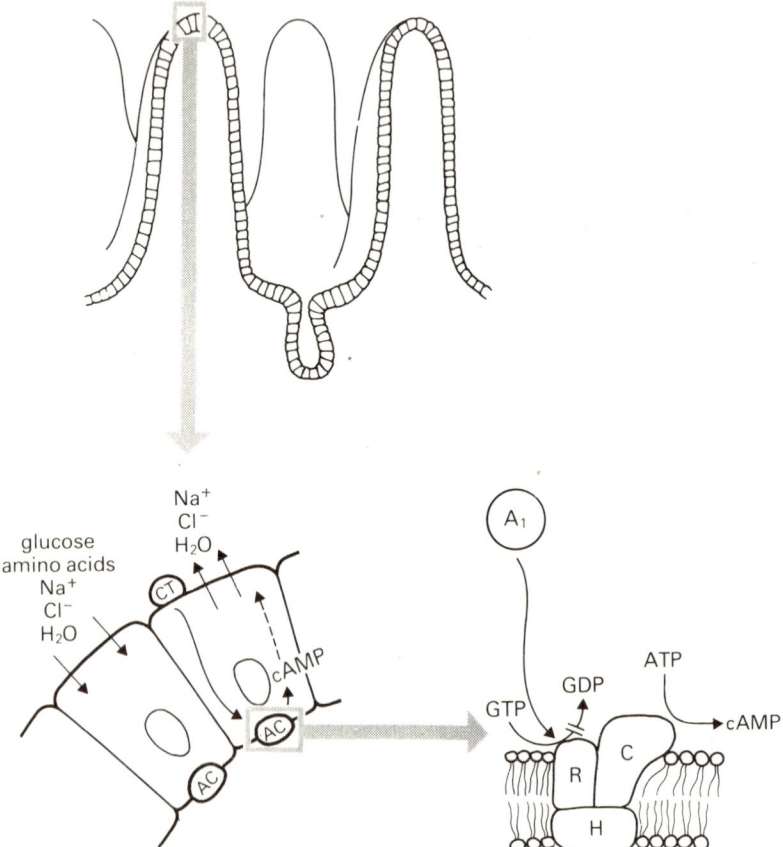

Figure 8 Mechanism by which cholera toxin causes diarrhoea. Binding of toxin to receptors on the lumen surface of ileal mucosal cells is followed by entry of fragment A_1, which interacts with the adenylate cyclase complex on the basal membrane, inhibiting the GTPase-mediated turn-off the cyclase (probably by ADP-ribosylation of the GTP-dependent regulator protein). Increased intracellular cyclic AMP levels cause, by some as yet unknown mechanism, efflux of Na^+ and Cl^- ions, and hence also water.

agreement with estimates of the number of adenylate cyclase complexes in pigeon erythrocytes. The target protein cannot be ADP-ribosylated by fragment A_1 from outside the cell, which strongly suggests that the site of ADP-ribosylation, and therefore in all probability, the site of adenylate cyclase activation, is intracellular. Thus, like diphtheria toxin, a portion of the whole toxin probably has to cross the cell membrane to exert its toxic activity. The fact that in the gut, cholera toxin binds to the mucosal surface of the epithelium, whereas adenylate cyclase activity resides in the basal surface requires such a process (Fig. 8).

The question we must now answer concerns the actual mechanism by which the A_1 fragment of cholera toxin stimulates adenylate cyclase activity. Adenylate cyclase has been recognized as a membrane-bound enzyme complex consisting of at least three components the nomenclature of which has yet to be unified: specific hormone receptors (H), situated on the outside of the membrane; a component (R) responsible for the GTP-dependent regulation of enzymic activity; and the component (C) responsible for the enzymic conversion of ATP to cyclic AMP. Both the regulatory and the enzymic components are situated on the inner surface of the cell membrane (see Fig. 8) and all three components may exist collectively as the adenylate cyclase complex or as individual proteins in the membrane.

It is thought that binding of a hormone to its receptor induces the binding of GTP to an active site on the regulatory component and that this brings about activation of the adenylate cyclase. This activation is turned off by hydrolysis of the bound GTP to give the inactive adenylate cyclase-GDP complex (Fig. 9). (It must be

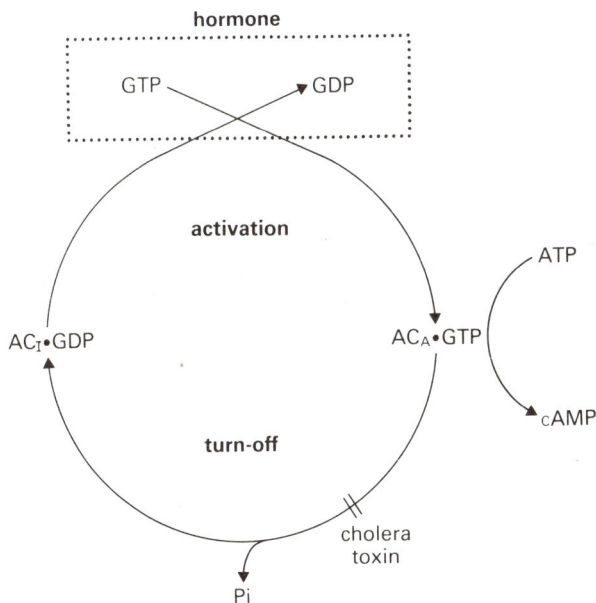

Figure 9 Proposed mechanism for the regulation of adenylate cyclase activity and site of action of cholera toxin (II). AC_A: activated adenylate cyclase; AC_I: inactive adenylate cyclase.

21

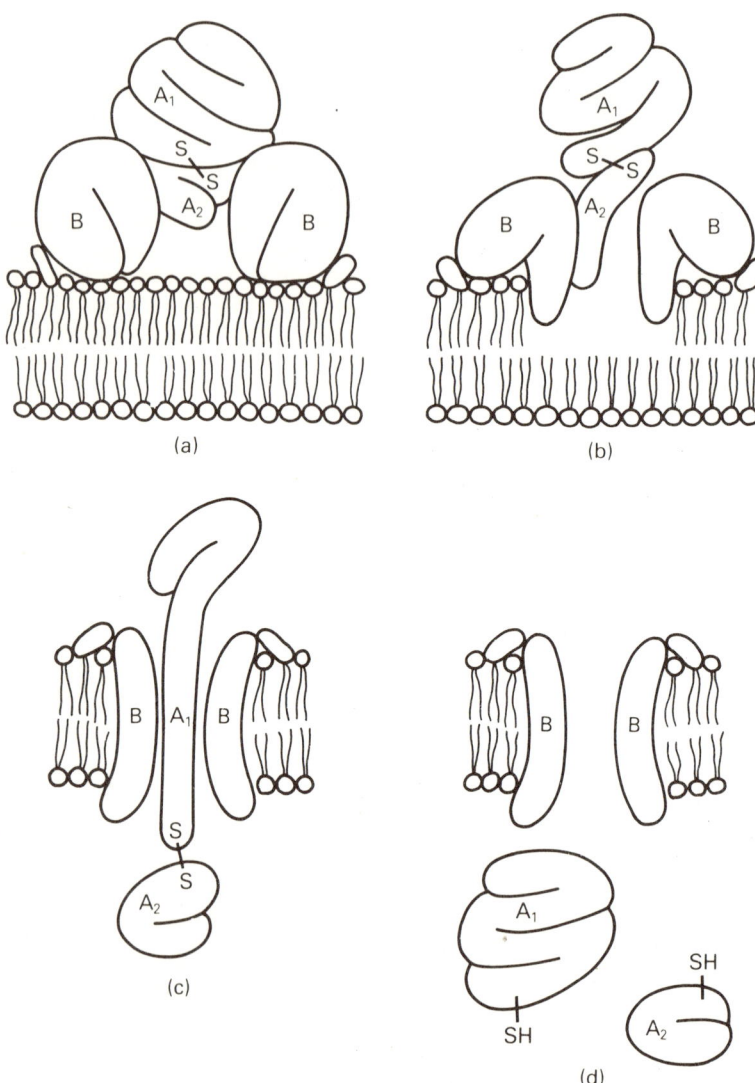

Figure 10 Proposed mechanism of entry of cholera toxin fragment A₁. Binding of B sub-units to specific receptors (a) induces a conformational change in these sub-units and their insertion into the membrane (b) to create a hydrophilic channel through which the A sub-unit can diffuse into the cell (c). Here, thiol agents reduce the disulphide bond, allowing fragment A₁ to diffuse into the cytoplasm and activate adenylate cyclase. (Reprinted with permission from Gill, D.M., *Biochemistry* (1976), **15**, 1242–1248.)

stressed at this stage, however, that cells exhibit low levels of adenylate cyclase activity even in the absence of hormones. It is this 'basal' activity that is stimulated by cholera toxin in lysed avian erythrocytes.)

Key evidence supporting this comes from Selinger's group in Israel who observed that hormone-induced activation of adenylate cyclase in the presence of the non-hydrolysable GTP analogue Gpp (NH) p is maximal and persistent, turn-off apparently being inhibited. It is important to note that Gpp (NH) p cannot activate adenylate cyclase in the absence of hormone; thus hormones appear to be responsible for the displacement of GDP from the regulatory site as well as the binding of GTP.

According to this concept of adenylate cyclase activation there are two possible ways in which cholera toxin could stimulate cyclase activity; it could enhance GTP association at the regulatory site or it could inhibit the GTPase turn-off reaction. Kinetic studies of cholera toxin-stimulated adenylate cyclase activity reveal that although the velocity constant for GTP association is unaffected by toxin, that of turn-off is drastically reduced, indicating that cholera toxin acts by inhibiting the GTPase turn-off reaction. If so, one would expect GTP to stimulate toxin-treated adenylate cyclase in the presence of hormone to the same extent as does Gpp (NH) p in the absence of toxin. This is indeed the case. Moreover, one can detect an inhibition of GTPase activity in toxin-treated membrane preparations which shows the same dependence upon toxin concentration as does adenylate cyclase activity.

Thus it is clear that cholera toxin fragment A_1 inhibits deactivation of hormone-stimulated adenylate cyclase by interfering with GTP hydrolysis at the regulatory site of the complex, almost certainly by ADP-ribosylation, and thereby increases levels of intracellular cyclic AMP, which by some as yet unknown mechanism evokes efflux of Na^+ and Cl^- and hence also of water. This suggestion becomes even more attractive in view of the observations by Gill that the target for ADP-ribosylation by A_1 in pigeon erythrocyte lysates is a protein of molecular weight $42-43\,000$ daltons, as is the regulatory component of the adenylate cyclase.

Mode of entry In 1976, Gill proposed the following mechanism for entry, which is consistent with all subsequent observations regarding the structure and activity of cholera toxin. Binding of the toxin to the cell is effected *via* the interaction of one B sub-unit and one molecule of ganglioside, or a similar molecule. Lateral diffusion of membrane gangliosides then enables receptors eventually to bind to all five B sub-units. The result of such binding is the localized increase in concentration of toxin at the cell surface, increasing the chances of subsequent penetration of the membrane by the A_1 fragment. This intimate interaction between the B region of the toxin and the cell membrane may be sufficient to allow A_1 to cross the membrane unaided, the B sub-units playing no further role in the entry process. However, an alternative hypothesis, taking account of the probable ring structure of the B region and the strong internal hydrophobic interactions of the B sub-units, is that these internal protein-protein forces are replaced by lipid-protein interactions, causing unfolding of the B sub-units to form a hydrophilic tunnel in the membrane through which the A sub-unit can diffuse. At some stage the disulphide bridge between fragments A_1 and A_2 is presumably cleaved and A_1 is then free to exert its enzymic action in the cytoplasm (Fig. 10).

Whether sub-unit A reaches the cytoplasm by itself or through a channel created by B, the polypeptide must enter in an unfolded state and refold before interacting with adenylate cyclase. The stability of A_1 to treatment with detergent suggests that this fragment is capable of undergoing such conformational changes without loss of activity.

Cholera toxin as an immunogen Whereas the other classical monotoxic diseases such as diphtheria and tetanus have been controlled by the prophylactic administration of specific toxoid, an effective means of conferring immunity to cholera has still to be validated under field conditions. *V. cholerae* was long thought not to produce a toxin because intravenous injection of either organisms or sterile culture filtrates did not cause cholera. Cholera toxin acts upon the cells of the ileal mucosa, and can only reproduce the symptoms of the disease when administered by an appropriate route—for example, by injection into ligated ileal segments.

It seems likely that immunological protection against cholera toxin may be achieved only by the stimulation of a specific secretory IgA response in the gut. This poses two important problems. First, although parenteral administration of antigen evokes a large humoral antibody response, it stimulates little localized secretory IgA response. Second, any secretory IgA response evoked is transient, usually lasting no longer than six months, and does not as far as is known confer any lasting immunological memory, so that several years after the initial immunological response the patient often has no more immunity to further challenge than someone receiving a primary challenge. Thus, the problems inherent in developing an immunizing regime for cholera are great. However, protective immunological responses need not be directed solely against the toxin, for although cholera toxin is responsible for all the symptoms of the disease it is not the sole virulence determinant of *V. cholerae*: the latter must adhere to and colonize the small intestine before causing diarrhoea. Indeed, toxigenic strains of *V. cholerae* which lack specific surface structures necessary for localization and colonization of the small intestine do not cause experimental cholera. Immunity to cholera may be achieved, therefore, by the stimulation of a localized immune response in the gut to cholera toxin and/or to the surface structures of *V. cholerae*.

Holmgren and Svennerholm in Sweden have shown that while parenteral (subcutaneous) administration of *V. cholerae* lipopolysaccharide (see Chapter 6), containing antigens important in adhesion, or enterotoxin to Swedish women stimulates a specific serum antibody response; the secretory IgA response of saliva and milk, which presumably reflects intestinal IgA levels, is only poorly stimulated. However, similar administrations of antigen to Pakistani women, whose milk and saliva often contain low levels of specific secretory IgA (presumably as a result of prior exposure to *V. cholerae*), significantly boost IgA levels, indicating that parenteral cholera vaccination may be effective in intestinally primed individuals.

It is the possibility of developing an orally administered cholera vaccine that is now undergoing most research. Lange and Holmgren reported, in 1978, that although repeated intravenous injections of cholera toxin do not protect mice against the diarrhoeagenic effects of cholera toxin as judged by the ileal loop test, repeated oral administration of toxin, while conferring no marked serum antitoxin titre, gives considerable protective immunity in the ileum. Others have obtained similar results with dogs. Thus the future for a cholera vaccine may depend upon the development of an orally administered antigen preparation which will stimulate long-lasting localized specific secretory IgA-mediated protection.

Finkelstein and his colleagues in Texas have recently isolated a variant of *V. cholerae* with a mutation in the gene for toxin production such that choleragenoid, but no A sub-unit, is synthesized freely. They hope that this variant, designated in true Texan fashion 'Texas Star', may be used as a live vaccine which, when administered orally, will colonize the ileum and release choleragenoid, so persistently stimulating a specific secretory IgA response. However, the usefulness of such a live vaccine depends on the organism's ability to persist in the small intestine and its inability to revert to toxigenicity.

Enterotoxins of *Escherichia coli*

It has long been known that certain strains of the biochemists' favourite bacterium, *E. coli*, can cause acute diarrhoea in man and animals. Recently the organism has been implicated in cases of clinical cholera. Enteropathogenic strains of *E. coli*, when injected into ligated ileal loops, behave like *V. cholera* in causing fluid accumulation, and this enterotoxic effect can be reproduced with cell-free preparations from culture fluids. Further work has revealed that most enteropathogenic strains of *E. coli* produce a heat-labile enterotoxin (LT) and sometimes also elaborate a distinguishable heat-stable enterotoxic factor (ST). The incidence of enteropathogenic *E. coli* producing ST alone is low but significant. Production of both toxins is mediated by transmissible plasmids and thus organisms carrying these plasmids may be able to transfer enterotoxigenicity to other Gram-negative bacterial species. This may explain the isolated reports of enterotoxin production by strains of *Salmonella, Yersinia*, and *Pseudomonas*.

The heat-labile enterotoxin (LT) of *E. coli* acts by stimulating adenylate cyclase activity and so, superficially at least, resembles cholera toxin. The extent to which LT resembles cholera toxin is not fully understood because workers have experienced great difficulty in preparing LT in pure, active form from culture filtrates. Different investigators have isolated heat-labile enterotoxic proteins of molecular weight varying between approximately 80 000 and 105 000 daltons. However, it has been shown that such preparations can be activated by treatment with trypsin, suggesting that LT may be synthesized as a high molecular weight polypeptide protoxin and that the enterotoxic form is a proteolytic cleavage product of this. Evidence for this comes from the observation that LT from the periplasmic space of enteropathogenic *E. coli* is of relatively low molecular weight.

LT is antigenically similar to cholera toxin in that antibodies prepared against either toxin cross-neutralize both toxic activities. LT must therefore possess a region that is antigenically similar to at least a portion of cholera toxin sub-unit B. As well as having characteristics of cholera toxin sub-unit B, *E. coli* LT appears to possess properties very similar to those of fragment A_1 of choleragen. Gill and colleagues have shown that the enterotoxic product released from the periplasmic space of *E. coli* not only has a molecular weight very similar to that of cholera toxin fragment A_1, but also that it activates adenylate cyclase in the pigeon erythrocyte lysate system by a mechanism that is very similar if not identical to that of A_1.

More recently, it has been reported that, like fragment A_1, LT possesses ADP-ribosylating activity. In fact, no important differences have been found between LT from the periplasmic space and A_1 and, therefore, it is tempting to assume that the two proteins are, if not identical, very closely related. Considerable support for this proposal has come from the genetic studies of Falkow's group in Seattle. They have cloned the smallest piece of plasmid DNA that will code for a functional heat-labile enterotoxic product. The latter has been generated in large quantities, immunoprecipitated with anti-LT serum and shown by electrophoresis of the dissociated immunoprecipitate to consist of two proteins, one of molecular weight 11 500 daltons (about the same size as cholera toxin sub-unit B) and the other of molecular weight approximately 25 500 daltons (similar to fragment A_1 and the periplasmic LT). The similarities between LT and cholera toxin are obviously great and suggest at least a common ancestor for these two toxins. Indeed, LT may differ functionally from cholera toxin only in its lack of a fragment A_2-like moiety.

The heat-stable enterotoxin (ST) of *E. coli* is very different from LT. It is non-antigenic and has a very low molecular weight (4 500–5 000 daltons). ST has recently been purified sufficiently for its mode of action to be studied *in vitro* and it has been found to be superficially similar to LT and cholera toxin in that it causes an increase in the short circuit current across stripped segments of rabbit ileal mucosa in an Ussing chamber. However, unlike LT and cholera toxin, this change is accompanied by an increase in cellular levels of cyclic GMP, rather than cyclic AMP. There are other obvious differences between the mode of action of ST and that of LT or cholera toxin. ST rapidly transmits its 'signal' across the membrane, producing a change in the activity of the cyclase that is readily reversible by dissociation of ST from the cell membrane. NAD^+ and cytosol proteins do not appear to be necessary for ST activity in lysed cell preparations.

Initially, doubts were cast that activation of guanylate cyclase could bring about changes in ion transport leading to diarrhoea, since insulin and cholecystokinin, two hormones known to activate guanylate cyclase, do not cause fluid accumulation in ligated ileal loops. However, recent reports suggest that addition of the stable analogue of cyclic GMP, 8-bromo-cyclic GMP, can cause fluid accumulation under similar conditions. Thus it is possible that ST does cause diarrhoea by activating guanylate cyclase in the intestinal mucosa. However it is likely that the mechanism of activation is more akin to that brought about by hormones than by other bacterial enterotoxins.

Role in pathogenesis Although from the evidence described here it is clear that the enterotoxins of *E. coli* are very important factors in the production of enteropathogenic lesions, they are by no means the only factors important in virulence. For example, the ability of a strain of *E. coli* to produce diarrhoea is, like *V. cholerae*, also dependent upon its ability to adhere to the mucosal surface of the intestine and thus to overcome mechanical clearance from the system by intestinal motility. Thus strains of *E. coli* lacking surface structures responsible for adhesion and colonization of the intestine do not cause diarrhoea even though they retain their ability to produce enterotoxin. Equally, strains of piglets which do not possess the mucosal receptors for the surface structures have been shown to be resistant to fully virulent *E. coli*.

Neurotoxins: tetanus and botulinum toxins

Although these two toxins cause disease syndromes that are usually quite dissimilar, they will be considered together here since their structural and functional similarities outweigh their dissimilarities.

Tetanus toxin Tetanus is an exceedingly unpleasant disease caused by wound infection by the anaerobe *Clostridium tetani* and characterized by severe painful spasms and rigidity of the voluntary muscles (a state of 'tetanus'). Development of disease is dependent upon the introduction and germination of spores of *C. tetani* in host tissue, but in clean and healthy wounds, although infection with spores may occur, germination and hence disease, is prevented by the aerobic conditions. If, however, the wound is necrotic or infected with other bacteria, the oxygen tension may be low enough to allow spores to germinate and cause disease. In such cases the tetanus victim experiences, usually some 7–10 days after infection, intermittent, mild muscular contractions at or near the site of the wound. These symptoms rapidly increase until the victim is wracked by violent convulsive spasms in the torso and limbs of a body contorted by generalized muscular contractions. These severe symptoms are frequently preceded or accompanied by spasm of the jaw muscles (trismus) which is why the disease is often referred to as 'lockjaw'. Death is inevitable and usually results from the victim's inability to control his or her breathing. What makes the disease especially distressing is the fact that the victim is conscious at all times and is only too aware of what is happening.

Although *C. tetani* also produces an oxygen-labile membrane damaging toxin, 'tetanolysin' (see Chapter 3), the pathogenicity of tetanus is based solely upon the effects of a powerful neurotoxin, (tetanus toxin, 'tetanospasmin'), which is elaborated by cells multiplying at the site of infection, where it interacts with the nervous system. The involvement of a toxin was first suggested in the late 1880s by Kitasato, who performed the first of the now classical 'point of no return' experiments, from which we can deduce the involvement of toxins in disease. Kitasato showed that mice injected in the tail with tetanus bacilli showed no ill-effects if the site of injection was excised within half an hour. If, however, excision was carried out at any time later than 30 min they developed tetanus and died even though organisms could not be isolated from the dead animals' tissues. The toxin exerts its action on the central reflex apparatus in the spinal cord, where it accumulates and causes continual excitation of the motor neurones by a mechanism described in more detail later.

Botulinum toxin *Clostridium botulinum* is widely distributed in the environment, spores being present in dust, soil, lake deposits, and on the surface of vegetation. For this reason, the intestinal contents may often contain spores of the organism. If foodstuffs* prepared from contaminated carcases are not properly cooked then, given favourable conditions, spores germinate and vegetative cells elaborate a powerful neurotoxin—together with tetanus toxin it is the most potent toxin known to man—which upon ingestion is absorbed through the intestine into the circulation and causes the disease known as botulism. Thus, classical human botulism was thought recently to differ from other microbial diseases in that it was not ordinarily considered to be an infectious disease, rather an intoxication. However, the work of several clinicians in California has radically changed this view. *C. botulinum* can grow in the intestines of babies and produce sufficient toxin to cause serious illness. Although hospitalized cases rarely prove fatal, it is believed that if severe infection occurs, then toxin production may rapidly lead to death of the infant; thus 'infant botulism' may be a cause of sudden infant death syndrome (SIDS or 'cot death' in developed countries is the most common cause of death among children aged 1 month to 1 year and estimated to claim 8–10 000 victims a year in the USA alone).

* Ermengen originally isolated organism from contaminated sausage (L., *botulus* = sausage).

Bacterial Toxins

To investigate this possibility Arnon and Midura recently obtained specimens of serum, tissue and bowel contents from infants under the age of one year who had died suddenly, and examined them for the presence of *C. botulinum* and toxin. Bacteria or toxin could be detected in nine of the 211 SIDS victims studied, but were found in only one of 69 infants who died of other causes. Thus, *C. botulinum* can cause an infectious disease which, in the state of California at least, may account for some sudden deaths in infants.

The first symptoms of botulism food poisoning—nausea, constipation, dizziness and severe dryness of the throat—usually develop between 12 and 36 hours after consumption of contaminated food. Obvious neurological disorders then develop, characterized by dilation of the pupils and blurred vision, difficulty in swallowing, general weakness and, finally, respiratory paralysis leading to death by asphyxia. The symptoms of infectious botulism in infants are essentially similar. All these symptoms are attributable to the neuro-pathological effect of botulinum toxin, which acts primarily at the neuromuscular junction, blocking stimulation of muscle contraction and thereby causing *flaccid* paralysis. In rare cases botulinum toxin, like tetanus toxin, may pass along motor nerve fibres to the spinal cord and there block neurotransmission.

Structure There is now reasonable agreement among workers in the field that tetanus and botulinum toxins are synthesized as single polypeptide chains of approximate molecular weight 150 000 daltons which, when released by bacteria, are proteolytically cleaved to a 'nicked' form of the toxin consisting of two non-identical protein fragments, designated A (approximately 50 000 daltons) and B (approximately 100 000 daltons), held together by a disulphide bond. There are thus structural similarities between the neurotoxins and diphtheria and other sub-unit toxins.

Fragment B of tetanus toxin is non-toxic and is capable of binding to susceptible cell membranes and will compete with whole toxin for specific binding sites (disialogangliosides, GD_2 and GD_{1b}; see Fig. 2). Fragment A is non-toxic to cells but is required for toxicity of the whole molecule. However, our limited knowledge of this fragment and the molecular basis of tetanus toxin action prevents direct comparison with A fragments of other toxins, though it is tempting to speculate that, on the basis of its structure, tetanus toxin has an intracellular site of action that depends upon some activity of the A fragment.

Although *C. botulinum* produces at least six distinct neurotoxins (A to F) which differ from each other in their immunological characteristics, relative toxicities, and the animal types normally affected (for latter see Table 1), their structures and biochemical action are essentially similar and, unless otherwise stated, the features of botulinum toxin to be described here are common to all types.

Studies of the structure and action of botulinum toxin have, until the last decade, been hampered because in crude form, the toxic product of *C. botulinum* consists of a complex of two distinct components: a haemagglutinin of molecular weight approximately 500 000 daltons and the neurotoxin (botulinum toxin) which, like tetanus toxin, has a molecular weight of approximately 150 000 daltons. The complex of haemagglutinin and neurotoxin is sometimes referred to as 'progenitor toxin' and the isolated neurotoxin as 'derivative toxin'. Recently Japanese workers have shown that progenitor toxin is more resistant to proteolysis and low pH than neurotoxin; thus the haemagglutinin component of the high molecular weight toxin complex appears to protect the neurotoxic component against inactivation in the

Table 1 *Clostridium botulinum* toxin serotypes and associated diseases.

Toxin	Animal species affected (disease)*	Source of intoxication
A	man chickens (limberneck)	home-preserved fruit and vegetables; meat; fish
B	man horses cattle infant botulism	meat infectious disease
C_α	water fowl (western duck disease)	greenfly larvae; rotting vegetation in ponds
C_β	cattle (midland cattle disease) horses (forage poisoning) mink	forage; carrion; pig liver
D	cattle (lamziekte)	carrion
E	man	uncooked seafood
F	man	meat produce

* Name given to specific disease syndrome in a particular animal species.

gut. Although no experimental evidence exists to support the view, most workers in the field feel that, in keeping with the general model for sub-unit toxin action, fragment B binds the toxin to nerve cells and fragment A is responsible for neurotoxic effects.

Modes of action Tetanus toxin acts primarily on the central reflex apparatus in the spinal cord, causing continual excitation of the motor neurones and hence spastic paralysis. Before explaining how the toxin effects these changes in the central nervous system, it is necessary briefly to familiarize readers with the essential features of muscle action (Figs. 11, 12). To do this the basic reflex arc system will be described for simplicity, although it must be stressed that tetanus toxin exerts its effects primarily upon the voluntary muscles.

All muscles are reciprocally innervated; that is to say, the contraction of a protagonist extensor muscle is inhibited by the contraction of its antagonist flexor muscle. Thus, in the reflex arc system, sensory afferent nerve fibres mediate both activation of protagonist muscle contraction and inhibition of antagonist muscle contraction. The sensory afferent neurone stimulates the motor neurone by secretion of the excitatory neurotransmitter acetylcholine (ACh) at the motor synapse. The motor neurone then triggers muscle contraction by secretion of ACh at the neuromuscular junction. It is known that different branches of a single nerve fibre always secrete the same neurotransmitter. How then, can another branch of the sensory afferent fibre also cause inhibition of antagonist muscle contraction, since the nerve endings must also secrete ACh?

Unlike stimulation of contraction, inhibition by an afferent neurone is indirect.

29

Bacterial Toxins

The neurone synapses with an inhibitory interneurone, stimulation of which leads to secretion of an inhibitory transmitter—glycine in the CNS, gamma-amino butyric acid (GABA) in the cerebellum—at the motor synapse, so abolishing stimulation of the motor neurone and hence muscle contraction. Therefore, to effect spastic paralysis of muscle, tetanus toxin must either increase the release of the stimulatory neurotransmitter ACh or abolish the effect or release of the inhibitory neurotransmitter glycine (or, less commonly, GABA); experimental evidence favours the latter. But how does the toxin become localized at this site? Tetanus toxin in the neuromuscular region binds to, and is taken up by, motor nerve endings and travels along the nerve trunk to the spinal cord, the primary target organ. It is transported to the spinal cord actually inside the axons, by a process known as intra-axonal retrograde transport. This can be demonstrated by immunological and autoradiographical techniques.

How does the toxin travel up the axons? The work of Stockel and his colleagues suggests that transport may involve, initially at least, the binding of tetanus toxin to gangliosides. This idea is supported by the observation that administration of

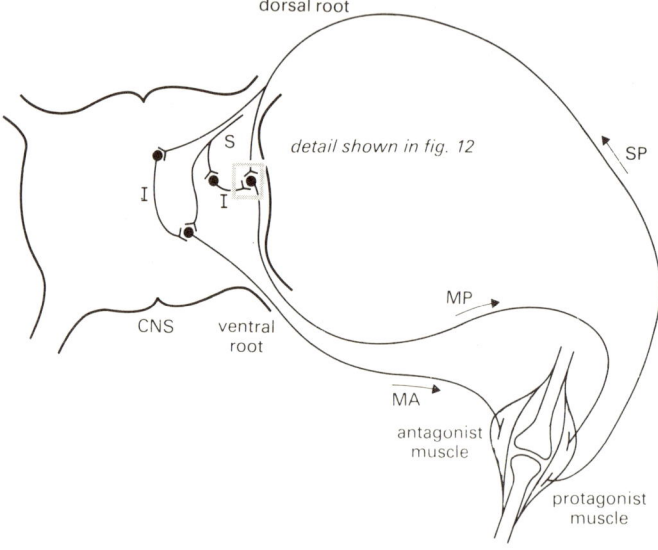

Figure 11 Mechanism for inhibiting the antagonists to a muscle contracting in response to stretch. Muscles are reciprocally innervated with sensory and motor neurones, although for clarity this is shown only for the protagonist muscle. On stretch, the stretch receptors generate an impulse which is transmitted along the afferent sensory (S) neurone (SP) of the protagonist muscle. This SP enters the spinal cord by the dorsal root and synapses with the motor neurone (MP) supplying the protagonist muscle and with an interneurone (I) which in turn synapses with the motor neurone (MA) supplying the antagonist muscle; the efferent motor neurones leave the spinal cord by the ventral root. At the SP/MP synapse an excitatory transmitter is released which induces an impulse in MP which leads to contraction of protagonist muscle. However, excitation of I causes release of an inhibitory transmitter at the I/MA synapse which leads to relaxation of the antagonist muscle. A simplified version of the biochemical events occurring in synapses is given in Fig. 12.

neuraminidase (an enzyme which degrades gangliosides) before that of tetanus toxin, blocks transport, as does pre-incubation of toxin with gangliosides. It has been suggested that the toxin binds to the gangliosides of GD_2 and GD_{1b} at the motor nerve ending and is then taken up into the axon by endocytosis and is transported within vesicles. Thus, the interaction between tetanus toxin and ganglioside may represent a necessary step in transport rather than a toxin-receptor interaction *per se* because binding of toxin to ganglioside does not necessarily lead to a toxic effect on that cell.

Following transport to the motor synapse, tetanus toxin then exerts its toxic effect, causing continual stimulation of the motor neurone. There is now good evidence that tetanus toxin acts presynaptically, affecting not the synthesis of the inhibitory neurotransmitter glycine, but its release into the synaptic cleft. The sensitivity of the motor neurone to glycine is unaffected by intoxication, the effects of which can be overcome *in vitro* by addition of glycine. The blockage of neurotransmitter release is not entirely restricted to glycine and GABA, however, as tetanus toxin in rare cases acts peripherally to block the release of ACh at the neuromuscular junction, so causing flaccid paralysis.

Thus, to exert its most common toxic effect, tetanus toxin must be released from the motor neurone, cross the synaptic cleft, and interact with the inhibitory neuronal endings; and there is evidence that this does take place. However, the

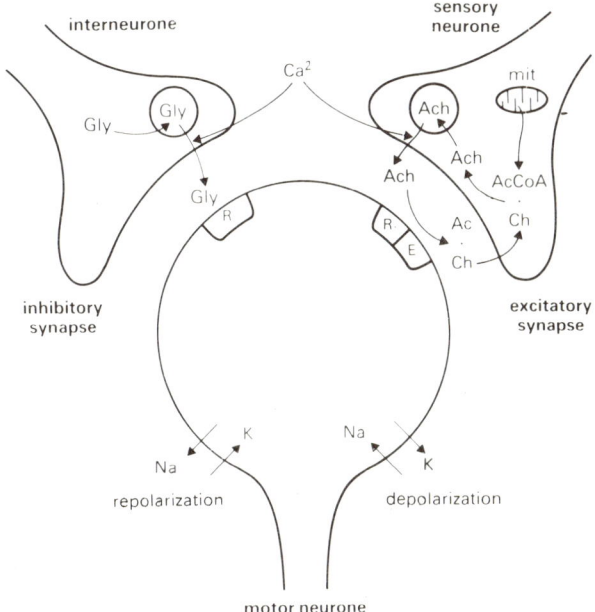

Figure 12 Excitatory and inhibitory synapses: neurotransmitter release and action. For a full description, see text.

Ac CoA: acetylcoenzyme A; ACh: acetylcholine; Ch: choline; Gly: glycine; R_1 and R_2: specific postsynaptic receptors for neurotransmitters;
E: acetylcholine esterase; mit: mitochondria.

31

mechanism by which tetanus toxin effects this complex passage and indeed the number of membranes that tetanus toxin must interact with and/or cross are under intense study.

Although it has long been known that botulinum toxin binds, apparently *via* gangliosides, to ACh–containing nerve endings, thereby inhibiting muscle contraction, the molecular mechanism of toxin action is still unknown. In order to put our limited knowledge into perspective, we will briefly describe what little is known about the physiology of cholinergic nerve endings, where it differs from that of inhibitory nerve endings described in the section on tetanus toxin. ACh is synthesized from choline and acetyl CoA by the action of the enzyme choline acetyltransferase and is then packaged into synaptic vesicles (Fig. 12). The invasion of a nervous impulse causes rapid influx of Ca^{2+} ions, which in some way causes efflux of ACh, presumably by exocytosis. ACh crosses the synaptic cleft and interacts with specific receptors on muscle or a nerve cell body, causing depolarization. The neurotransmitter then either diffuses away or undergoes esteric cleavage to acetate and choline, which is taken up by the nerve ending for the resynthesis of ACh.

In accordance with this model, botulinum toxin may cause flaccid paralysis in two ways: inhibition of ACh synthesis either by inhibition of choline acetyltransferase, or by blockage of choline uptake from the synaptic cleft, or by inhibition of ACh release. The evidence points to the latter as the mechanism of action of botulinum toxin. Thus, like tetanus toxin, botulinum toxin acts presynaptically to block neurotransmitter release. Indeed, in primary rat nerve cell cultures, the effects of the two toxins are qualitatively identical, both blocking ACh release.

The molecular mechanism of inhibition of neurotransmitter release Our knowledge of the mechanisms by which both toxins block neurotransmitter release is scant, but reveals significant similarities between the two toxins. Neurotransmitters are believed to be synthesized in the region of the nerve endings and packaged into synaptic vesicles. Release occurs by exocytosis of the synaptic vesicle or its contents and appears to be dependent upon the increase of the axoplasmic Ca^{2+} concentration during nervous impulse transmission (see Fig. 12). Synaptosomal membrane fractions contain actin and synaptic vesicles are coated with myosin: neurotransmitter release may thus involve contact between vesicles and presynaptic membranes with the formation of an actomyosin-like protein (AMLP) possessing Ca^{2+}–dependent ATPase activity. In the presence of Ca^{2+}, ATP hydrolysis could cause contraction of AMLP, inducing a change in the synaptic vesicles and secretion of neurotransmitter into the synaptic cleft. Tetanus toxin has been shown to bind to AMLP, decreasing contractile ability by inhibition of Ca^{2+}–dependent ATPase activity. Thus, tetanus toxin may block inhibitory neurotransmitter release by inhibiting the contraction of AMLP and subsequent exocytosis of synaptic vesicles of their contents.

It has also been suggested that tetanus toxin might act by affecting cyclic nucleotide metabolism. In toxin-induced paralysis of the iris, a temporary reversal of toxin effect by cyclic nucleotides and by theophylline, an inhibitor of phosphodiesterase (cyclic nucleotide antagonist) activity, is observed. Certainly cyclic nucleotides seem to play an important role in synaptic transmission, probably by maintaining synaptic vesicle integrity, and may be involved in Ca^{2+} uptake by synaptic terminals, so alteration of cyclic nucleotide metabolism by tetanus toxin could influence inhibitory neurotransmitter release.

Recently, work has been carried out in London by Wonnacott and co-workers on the molecular basis for the inhibition of neurotransmitter release by botulinum toxin. Pre-incubation of isolated synaptosomes from guinea pig cerebral cortex with botulinum toxin causes an inhibition of ACh release upon depolarization which can be overcome either by raising the extracellular Ca^{2+} concentration or by treatment of the synaptosomes with ionophore A 23187, which allows Ca^{2+} ions to cross membranes freely. Thus, botulinum toxin in some way interferes with the supply, or action, of Ca^{2+}, the influx of which is necessary for ACh release. Whether the toxin effects these changes from the cell surface or intracellularly, which would fit our general concept of sub-unit toxin action, is still unknown.

Simpson, in 1974, produced evidence to support an intracellular site of action. He showed that toxin-induced paralysis is at least a two-step process involving initial binding of toxin to the nerve ending which is independent of temperature, is poorly reversible, and which can be antagonized by antitoxin. A second step is dependent upon temperature, neurotransmitter release (perhaps to expose sites at which the toxin acts), is irreversible and, most importantly, cannot be antagonized by antitoxin. This resembles the mechanics of interaction of diphtheria toxin with susceptible cells, where initial binding is followed by an internalization process which is dependent upon the fluidity of the cell membrane, and hence temperature, and which cannot be inhibited by antitoxin, since whole toxin is no longer localized at the cell surface.

Most workers believe, albeit without any good evidence, that, like other toxins described in this chapter, tetanus and botulinum toxins have an intracellular site of action. But is this action enzymic? Habermann and Dimpfel, in 1973, estimated the concentration of tetanus toxin in the spinal cord of intoxicated animals to be approximately 10^{-15} M which to some seems to preclude any mechanism other than an enzymic one for tetanus toxin action. In contrast however, Hanig and Lamanna recently postulated a stoichiometric model for botulinum toxin, based on estimates of the number of botulinum toxin molecules reaching an intoxicated neuromuscular end-plate and the number of ACh containing vesicles and sites for ACh release.

Colicins E3 and E2

Certain coliform bacteria produce toxic proteins with properties similar to those of toxins already described in this chapter but which exert their toxic action not on eukaryotic cells, but on other related strains of bacteria.

Colicin E3 is elaborated by coliform bacteria carrying the plasmid Col E3. Specific binding of the colicin to susceptible cells is followed, after a short lag phase, by rapid inhibition of protein synthesis, caused by cleavage of a 50-nucleotide fragment (thought to interact with mRNA during initiation) from the 3′ end of 16S ribosomal RNA in intact ribosomes. Thus the colicin has an intracellular site of action.

Organisms carrying the Col E3 plasmid are immune to colicin E3. This immunity differs from the resistance shown by unrelated species, which lack colicin binding sites, in that it is due to the synthesis of an acidic protein also coded by the plasmid. This protein, called E3 immunity protein, binds to the colicin and thus prevents ribosomal inactivation.

Purified colicin E3 comprises a 50 000-dalton component, called E3* or protein

A, and the 10 000-dalton immunity protein. Protein A is more active in cell-free protein synthesizing systems than colicin E3 but possesses no bactericidal activity, suggesting that, as well as protecting colicinogenic cells against protein A, the immunity protein is involved in binding colicin to susceptible cells. Thus, the structure-function relationships of colicin E3 appear to be similar to those of cholera toxin in that they consist of a binding protein (immunity protein) non-covalently attached to a polypeptide (protein A) which apparently interacts with the susceptible cell membrane in such a way that it, or a proteolytic fragment of it, is released into the cytoplasm where it exerts its toxic action. The entry mechanism must differ from that for cholera toxin since the colicin must also traverse the bacterial cell wall. However, it has been suggested that receptors, which are probably glycoproteins, may be located at points where the cell wall and membrane are in intimate contact, thus facilitating entry.

Another colicin that has an apparent intracellular site of action is E2, which exhibits deoxyribonuclease activity *in vitro*.

Similar proteins of non-bacterial origin

The toxic lectins, abrin and ricin Although plant lectins (defined as proteins capable of binding to and agglutinating animal cells) are not usually toxic, certain lectins, of which the best known and most studied are abrin (from the seeds of the tropical legume *Abrus precatorius*) and ricin (found in castor seeds, *Ricinus communis*), are among the most toxic substances known. They are proteins of approximate molecular weight 65 000 daltons and consist of two individually non-toxic polypeptide moieties, designated fragments A and B, held together by a disulphide bond. The intracellular target for these lectins is the 60S ribosomal sub-unit, which is enzymically modified by an, as yet, unknown mechanism such that EF1- and EF2-dependent GTP hydrolysis is severely reduced, so inhibiting protein synthesis. The target site appears to be identical with, or in very close proximity to, the EF2 binding site on the ribosome, since pre-bound EF2 protects ribosomes against inactivation.

Animal glycoprotein hormones The pituitary glycoprotein hormones—thyrotropin (TSH), lutotropin (LH), follitropin (FSH), and human choriogonadotropin (HCG)—consist of two dissimilar polypeptide chains designated a sub-unit and β sub-unit, held together by non-covalent forces. Whereas the amino acid sequences of the different β sub-units differ markedly, the a-sub-unit of each hormone appears to be essentially identical. Thus it has been suggested that the β sub-units confer tissue specificity while the a-sub-units are at least, in part, responsible for the common action of these hormones (that is, activation of adenylate cyclase).

In view of the structural similarities between the glycoprotein hormones and the bacterial sub-unit toxins, many (though not all) workers have postulated that the β-sub-units are analogous to toxin B fragments, that they are responsible for binding to specific receptors on cell surfaces and facilitate the entry of the a-sub-unit into the cytoplasm where it can act. Although there is no formal proof that the glycoprotein hormones act by a mechanism similar to that of bacterial sub-unit toxins, and in particular cholera toxin, our current knowledge of the structure and properties of these proteins is not inconsistent with such a mechanism of action. For a recent review of this situation see Neville and Ta-min Chang (1978).

Summary

Six bacterial toxins consist of two types of sub-unit which, where characterized, are designated A and B: diphtheria (DT), *Psuedomonas aeruginosa* exotoxin A (PsT), cholera (CT), *Escherichia coli* heat-labile (LT), botulinum (BoT), and tetanus (TeT) toxins.

The B sub-units of DT and CT attach to receptors on susceptible cell membranes and somehow facilitate the intracytoplasmic uptake of the active A sub-unit; similar mechanisms are inferred for LT and PsT. DT and PsT inhibit host-protein synthesis; CT and LT elevate levels of cAMP in ileal epithelial cells resulting in imbalanced ion-transport and diarrhoea. DT, PsT, CT and LT possess a similar primary biochemical mode of action; that is, they catalyse the cleavage of NAD^+ and the transfer of ADPR to GTPase target proteins. In the case of DT and PsT the target is EF2 and for CT and LT it is the regulator protein in the adenylate cyclase complex.

P. aeruginosa also produces exoenzyme S, of as yet unproven relevance in infection, which ADP-ribosylates an unidentified substrate. *E. coli* heat-stable toxin (ST) is of low molecular weight, diarrhoeagenic, elevating intracellular guanylate cyclase levels.

At present, one can only speculate that BoT and TeT A and B sub-units have analogous functions to those of the other toxins. Current evidence suggests a similar primary mode of action for BoT and TeT; that is, interference with the normal influx of Ca^{2+} across presynaptic membranes. This results in the inhibition of exocytosis of excitatory (BoT) and inhibitory (TeT) neurotransmitters.

Other proteins which fall into this A–B sub-unit category include colicins E2 and E3, abrin and ricin, and animal glycoprotein hormones.

References

COLLIER, R. J. (1975). 'Diphtheria toxin: mode of action and structure.' *Bact. Rev. 39*: 54.

CUATRECASAS, P. Ed. (1976). 'The specificity and action of animal, bacterial and plant toxins.' In: *Receptors and recognition*, Series B, Vol. 1. Chapman and Hall. (Articles by B. Bizzini and L. L. Simpson on 'Tetanus toxin structure as a basis for elucidating its immunological and neurological activities' (p. 177) and 'Presynaptic actions of botulinum toxin and β-bungarotoxin' (p. 273).

DALLAS, W. S. & FALKOW, S. (1979). 'The molecular nature of heat-labile enterotoxin (LT) of *Escherichia coli*.' *Nature 277*: 406.

GILL, D. M. (1978). 'Seven toxic peptides that cross membranes.' In: *Bacterial toxins and cell membranes* p. 291. Edited by J. Jeljascewicz and T. Wadström. Academic Press.

NEVILLE, D. M. & CHANG, Ta-Min. (1978). 'Receptor-mediated protein transport into cells. Entry mechanisms for toxins, hormones, antibodies, viruses, lysosomal hydrolases, asialo-glycoproteins, and carrier proteins. In: *Current topics in membranes and transport 10*: 65. Edited by F. Bronner and A. Kleinzeller. Academic Press.

RODBELL, M. (1980). 'The role of hormone receptors and GTP-regulatory proteins in membrane transduction' *Nature 284*: 17.

SIMPSON, L. L. (1978). 'Pharmacological studies on the subcellular site of action of botulinum toxin type A.' *J. Pharmacol. and Exp. Ther. 206*: 661.

WONNACOTT, S., MARCHBANKS, R. M., & FIOL, C. (1978) 'Ca^{2+} uptake by synaptosomes and its effect on the inhibition of acetylocholine release by botulinum toxin.' *J. Neurochemistry 30*: 1127.

3 Membrane-damaging toxins; primary event defined

In the next two chapters we shall consider a group of toxins which damage cell membranes but whose roles in disease production have not been unequivocally established, possibly for several reasons.

First, the probable multifactorial nature of virulence of the pathogens producing the toxins creates difficulties in identifying and in ranking the importance of determinants of pathogenicity. In the case of gas gangrene and staphylococcal infections, powerful toxins are produced (at least *in vitro*) by the causative organisms together with a plethora of additional toxins, extracellular enzymes, and other factors of potentially comparable or perhaps co-operative relevance in pathogenicity.

Second, much of the experimental pathology of gas gangrene was determined when protein chemistry, in particular separation technology, was primitive by today's standards. The recognition of clostridial toxins relied upon crude protein fractionation methods allied to brilliant serology and the development of appropriate biological test systems. The demonstration of, say, lethal activity A in a complex culture filtrate containing other lethal factors required an antiserum containing antibodies to all lethal factors except A. The production of the requisite antisera was often only possible initially when strains were fortuitously isolated (or changed after isolation to those) which produced a different spectrum of antigens and hence elicited a correspondingly different spectrum of antibodies. The situation was further complicated when, as sometimes turned out to be the case, one antigen shared properties with other components in the same filtrate.

Third, most recent studies on membrane-damaging toxins have been carried out using highly purified materials, but with an emphasis on their cytotoxic and/or cytolytic effects *in vitro* rather than lethal or other effects *in vivo*. In this context much work has been done on red blood cells, even though haemolysis is rarely ever a feature of the diseases caused by the pathogens which elaborate these toxins: erythrocytes are convenient to obtain and handle in large quantities, and possess an inbuilt indicator system to demonstrate membrane damage when it occurs. Other cell systems, in particular leucocytes, have also been increasingly studied.

Thelestam, Mollby and Waström in Sweden have studied membrane damage by following the release of radio-labelled marker molecules of different sizes. By this means estimates of the functional size of the pores created by membrane-active substances can be obtained. In addition, naturally derived membrane vesicles or artificial phospholipid vesicles (liposomes) have been used. From such studies extrapolations could be made to what might happen when such toxins are elaborated in sub-lethal quantities *in vivo*. To some, but by no means all, this is an arguably superior approach to the toxinology of bacterial infections, especially in the context of non-lethal diseases caused by toxigenic pathogens.

The ensuing two chapters comprise a heterogeneous collection of toxins whose common feature is that they damage cell membranes. They bifurcate at the point which divides current biochemical knowledge and ignorance. Here we follow Freer and Arbuthnott, who recently grouped such toxins into those for which the most significant event in membrane interactions is defined and those for which comparable information is not yet available. In addition, we shall outline several considerations which hopefully will enrich the readers' appreciation of some complex interactive situations and of the difficulties in resolving them.

In this chapter we consider toxic molecules which destroy or derange known constituents of membranes leading to membrane disfunction and/or physical disruption. From the introductory chapter it is obvious that both proteins and lipids could constitute the target of toxin attack. We will not discuss the action of bacterial proteolytic enzymes because there is no good evidence to suggest that they play an important role (at least in the context of pathogenicity) in membrane damage. Proteolytic enzymes are involved, however, in destroying connective tissue. There are, however, many bacterial phospholipases which are capable of attacking membrane phospholipids. Another group of proteins, thiol-activated cytolysins, interact with cholesterol in the membrane while others have a detergent-like action on membranes.

Historically, the first toxin for which the biochemical mode of action was elucidated was the α-toxin produced by *Clostridium perfringens*. It is without doubt the most important toxin, from a disease-producing point of view, in this biochemical group. For these reasons phospholipases will be discussed first, with *C. perfringens* α-toxin as the example examined in greatest detail.

Phospholipase activity

Clostridium perfringens (*welchii*) α-toxin   The clostridial genus is one of the most prolific toxin-producing genera and *C. perfringens* one of the most toxigenic species in this group. By itself, or in concert with other species (these include *C. novyi, C. septicum, C. histolyticum*), it is the causative organism of gas gangrene which, though relatively rare except in warfare, is a rapid killer if not treated promptly: in fact, infections of man by histotoxic anaerobic bacteria are among the most acute and lethal known. For a masterly review the student is referred to Maclennan (1962).

Gas gangrene results from the contamination of deep muscle wounds by soil containing clostridial spores. The latter germinate in the complex conditions found in such an environment, in particular low Eh and pH*. Vegetative growth occurs and toxins are produced which kill the immediately surrounding tissues, thereby creating favourable conditions for the further spread of the organism. The extent of microbial invasion depends on the strain of the organism. From within this initial necrotic focus more toxin(s) is generated which diffuses into the rest of the body, producing toxaemia, a state of profound shock, and ultimately death. Dissemination of toxin must occur since loss or destruction of muscle *per se* will not cause death, certainly not rapid death, and early amputation of the affected limb is a highly effective treatment. Early administration of antibiotics and/or antitoxin

---

* This is an oversimplification; gas gangrene is a clinical entity. We do not know all of the precise conditions which predispose towards such a condition. It is possible to demonstrate wound contamination without overt clinical symptoms.

Table 2 Extracellular toxins and other products produced by Clostridial species

Species	Major lethal antigens; additional biological properties	Other antigens; biological properties	Type-specific groupings; some diseases
C. perfringens	α : phospholipase C, dermonecrotic, haemolytic. β : dermonecrotic ε : dermonecrotic produced as protoxin i : dermonecrotic	γ : lethal, non-haemolytic δ : lethal, haemolytic η : lethal, non-haemolytic θ : lethal, SH-activated cytolysin κ : lethal, collagenase λ : non-lethal, gelatinase μ : hyaluronidase ν : DNAse fibrinolysin.	A : α — gas gangrene (man); food poisoning (man) B : α, β, ε — lamb dysentery C : α, β. — Struck (sheep); necrotic enteritis (man) D : α, ε. — enterotoxaemia (sheep) E : α, i. — associated with disease of sheep, cattle; pathogenicity doubtful
C. novyi	α : dermonecrotic, produces extensive gelatinous oedema.	β : lethal, phospholipase C, dermonecrotic, haemolytic γ : phospholipase C, haemolytic δ : SH-activated cytolysin ε : lipase (not phospholipase C) ζ : haemolytic η : tropomyosinase θ : produces opalescence in egg-yolk	A : α, γ, ε. — gas gangrene (man; big head (rams) B : α, β, ζ, η. — gas gangrene (man); black disease (sheep) D : β, η, θ. — red water disease (cattle)
C. septicum	α : dermonecrotic, haemolytic, leucocidic, antigenically related to α -toxins of C. histolyticum and C. chauvoei	β : DNAse γ : hyaluronidase δ : SH-activated cytolysin	gas gangrene (man); braxy (sheep)

Species	Toxins	Toxins	Disease
C. histolyticum	α : dermonecrotic (see *C. septicum* α -toxin)	β : collagenase γ : SH-activated proteinase, haemolytic δ : non-SH-activated elastase ε : SH-activated cytolysin A total of 9 different proteolytic enzymes known	gas gangrene (man)- often associated, rarely the only causative organism
C. chauvoei	α : dermonecrotic, haemolytic. only slightly lethal, produced as part of soluble-immunizing component. (see *C. septicum* α -toxin)	β : DNAse γ : hyaluronidase δ : SH-activated cytolysin oedema factor soluble-immunizing-component insoluble-immunizing-component neuraminidase	black quarter (sheep, cattle)
C. sordelli, (*C. bifermentans;* closely related)	β : oedema producing, dermonecrotic (Greek symbols not widely used. Here we follow L. D. S. Smith, 1975)	α : phospholipase C (related to *C. perfringens* α-toxin) γ : proteinase SH-activated cytolysin phospholipase A, haemorrhagic factor (ex. sporulating cells)	gas gangrene (man)

This table is not exhaustive with respect to the number of toxigenic clostridial species, the number of toxins and other factors produced by each species, or the diseases for which they are the causative agents. Data compiled from *Principles of Bacteriology and Immunity* by Topley and Wilson; *The Pathogenic Anaerobic Bacteria* by L.D.S. Smith (Thomas; Springfield, Ill., 1975) and *Pathogenic Clostridia* by M. Sterne and I. Batty (Butterworth; London and Boston, 1975).

is also effective in preventing experimental gas gangrene. What, then, does *C. perfringens* produce that could account for the lethal infections it establishes?

From the early 40s to late 50s Oakley and his colleagues elucidated the biological nature of several extracellular toxins and antigens of potential relevance in disease production (Table 2). Modern immunoelectrophoretic analyses reveal many more soluble antigens secreted by this organism, but the vast majority remain as unidentified immunoprecipitates in gels. Despite this, we do know that type A strains, which cause human gas gangrene, produce only one lethal toxin in significant quantity. For this reason attention has been fixed on the elucidation of its nature and on the establishment of its presumptive role in causing this disease.

Nature of *Clostridium perfringens* α-toxin The toxin may first be formed as an inactive protoxin which is converted to the active form by Zn^{2+} ions. Biologically, α-toxin is lethal, necrotizing (it will cause localized destruction of skin tissue when injected intradermally in sub-lethal doses), and haemolytic. The correlations between the neutralization of all three activities by antisera and repeated failure to separate the activities even by most powerful techniques show that the three activities are due to a single species. In fact, highly purified α-toxin has repeatedly been electrofocused into three-to-five physicochemically distinct molecular species, but no one has ever separated the known biological activities associated with α-toxin. Neither the origin nor the significance of these molecular forms is known. However, they are most likely to represent post-translational modifications of the molecule. There is no evidence to support the suggestion that the multiplicity of molecular forms observed for an increasing number of toxins is the toxin equivalent of isoenzymes, so we do not propose to adopt the recently proposed term 'isotoxin'.

The first clue to its biochemical mode of action came independently, in 1939, from Seiffert in Germany and Nagler in Australia, who observed that sterile culture filtrates produced opalescence in normal human serum. Two years later, MacFarlane (RG), Oakley and Anderson observed that culture filtrates caused an intense turbidogenic reaction in sterile extracts of egg yolk. Serological analysis implicated a single factor as being responsible for the turbidogenic effects, the lysis of sheep red blood cells, and lethality. All these activities were Ca^{2+} dependent and, they concluded, due to α-toxin.

In the same year, MacFarlane (MG) and Knight formally proved that α-toxin enzymically releases phosphorylcholine and a neutral diglyceride from pure phosphatidyl choline (lecithin) and from the lipoproteins in egg yolk extracts and is thus a phospholipase C (Fig. 13). Thus for *the first time* an enzymic mechanism was assigned to a bacterial toxin. Later it was shown (see Table 3) that although phosphatidyl choline was the preferred substrate, as judged by the rate of hydrolysis, α-toxin would attack other phospholipids. Phospholipase activity is thus the common denominator linking various biological activities, which are different secondary *sequelae* to the same primary reaction. Turbidity in serum and egg-yolk extracts results from hydrolysis of phosphatidyl choline, destroying the structure responsible for stable micellar formations in lipoproteins, and producing a phase separation of lipid-rich materials. Haemolysis is preceded by release of phosphorylcholine from red cell membranes and is of the 'hot-cold' variety; that is, more lysis occurs when treated cells are cooled after incubation at 37°C; the phenomenon is discussed below in connection with staphylococcal β-haemolysin which provides the best example of this effect. The necrotic and lethal effects arise from the wide distribution of phosphatidyl choline in animal cell membranes, whose functional if not structural integrity would be impaired by hydrolysis of one of their major constituents.

The role of α-toxin in infection Since many cases of gas gangrene are caused by *C. perfringens* Type A on its own (although we must remember that some are of complex bacterial aetiology) which produces mainly α-toxin among the recognized major lethal toxins, attention was focused on the role that it played in the disease.

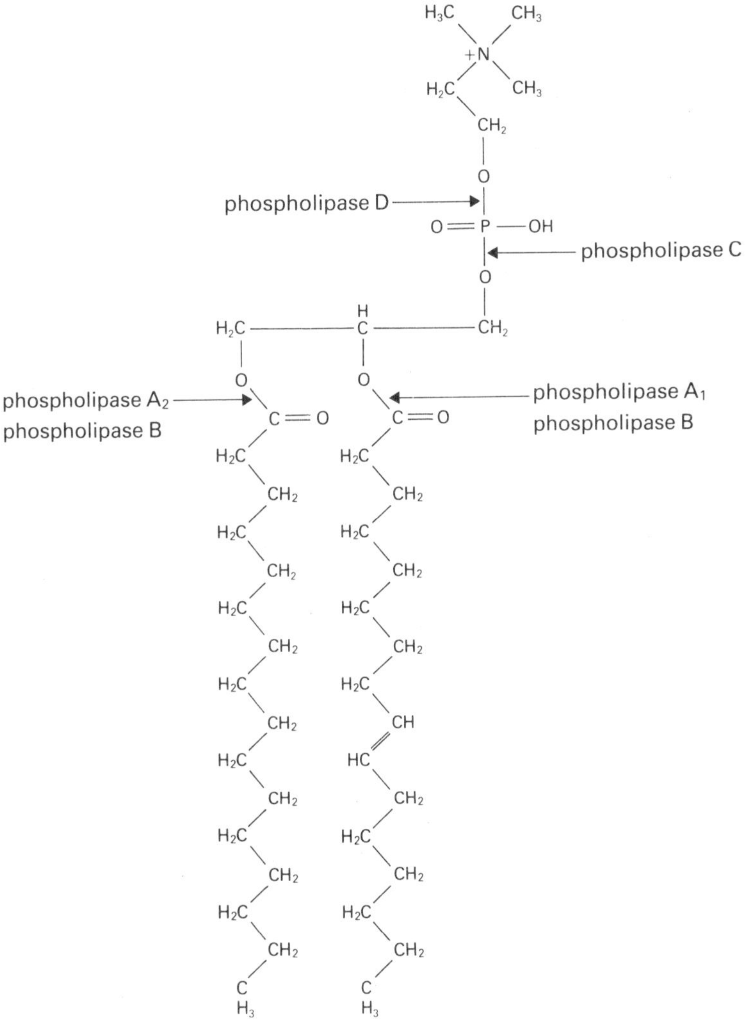

Figure 13 Sites of action of phospholipases. Sphingomyelinase C and D act at positions C and D respectively in sphingomyelin.

Table 3 Substrate specificities of, and antigenic relationships between, some bacterial phospholipases

Species	Enzyme/toxin	Antigenically related to	Substrate[1] Sph	PC	PE	PS	PI	L_{PE}^{PC}	PG	DPG	OPG
Clostridium perfringens	α-toxin	*C. bifermentans* enzyme	+[2]	+	+,	+	−[3]	+	−	−	−
C. novyi type A.	γ-toxin		+⁻	++	+	+	+	+			
C. novyi types B & D	β-toxin			++	+	+	+	+			
C. bifermentans		*C. perfringens* α-toxin	+	+							
C. sordellii	α-toxin	*C. perfringens* α-toxin									
Bacillus cereus	enzyme 1		−	+	+	+	−	+	+	+	+
Bacillus cereus	enzyme 2		−	−	−	−	+	+			
Staphylococcus aureus	β-haemolysin sphingomyelinase C		+	−	−	−	−	−	−	−	−
	enzyme 2		−	−	−	−	+	+	−	−	−
Pseudomonas aeruginosa			+	+	+	(+)[4]		+			
P. fluorescens			−	+	++	−	−	(+)	(+)	(+)	
P. aureofaciens				+	+	−	−	+	−	−	
Acinetobacter calcoaceticus			+	+	+	+					
Streptococcus hachijoensis			+	+	(+)	(+)	+	+		+	
Corynebacterium ovis	sphingomyelinase D		++								

1 Sph: sphingomyelin; PC: phosphatidyl choline; PE: phosphatidyl ethanolamine; PS: phosphatidyl serine; PI: phosphatidyl inositol; L_{PE}^{PC}: lysophosphatidyl choline or ethanolamine; PG: phosphatidyl glycerol; DPG: diphosphatidylglycerol; OPG: O-lysylphosphatidyl glycerol. Absolute comparisons are difficult in this context, since susceptibility to hydrolysis is determined by presence of specific cations and/or added solvents or detergents to promote enzyme-lipid interaction. The accessibility of substrate to enzyme and its rate of hydrolysis will also be determined by whether the substrate is in a dispersed or micellar form, or an integral part of a cell-membrane.

2 + = hydrolysed 3 − = not hydrolysed 4 (+) = weakly hydrolysed.

Information on substrate specificity reproduced with permission from Möllby, R. (1978). In *Bacterial Toxins and Cell Membranes* p. 367, ed. by

Was it involved, with or without the activities of the other factors listed in Table 2, in the generation of the local lesion and or the generalized toxaemia? The presence of gross oedema—so characteristic of this disease—signified changes in the permeability of capillaries which could be due to α-toxin acting on cell membranes. Histological examination of the lesion in man shows evidence of released fat globules (α-toxin), destruction of collagen fibrils (κ), loss of intercellular cement (μ), an absence of fibrin (fibrinolysin) deposition of which is a usual response to infection, and a lack of healthy leucocytes (α, γ and θ), which could be ascribed to the effects of the toxins in parentheses.*

Most of these features can be reproduced by exposing fresh excised muscle to sterile culture filtrates of *C. perfringens* type A, the principal exceptions being oedema and gas production, which are due to the host and the organism respectively and are probably important in aiding the spread of infection by opening up tissues. Despite these observations there is no consensus as to the importance and precise role of α-toxin in causing gas gangrene. The following brief discussion, using criteria outlined in Chapter 1 as guidelines, provides the student with a classic example of how difficult it is in some cases to pin down the microbial determinants of pathogenicity.

First, Evans in the early 1940s showed that for 25 out of 30 strains of *C. perfringens* type A there was a positive correlation between virulence in guinea pigs (used in many studies in experimental gas gangrene despite criticism by Oakley and others who have questioned their suitability because their thin muscle mass enhances the opportunity for invasion by the organisms) and ability to produce α-toxin, albeit in arbitrarily selected media. However, three avirulent strains produced toxin at levels which were at least equal to those of some virulent strains, and two strains produced very little toxin but showed a degree of virulence comparable to the group of toxigenic strains. Clearly it is the phenotype expressed *in vivo* and not *in vitro* that is important.

Second, the therapeutic value of antitoxic sera (containing a spectrum of antibodies but usually selected for high α-antitoxin levels) has been widely investigated in animals. In nearly every case, provided sera are given prophylactically or soon after infection in guinea pigs and sheep, the animals were protected against a lethal challenge with *C. perfringens*. The major exception comes from Bullen who, in a series of studies with guinea pigs, showed that successful antitoxic therapy was dependent largely on the method used for creating the tissue damage necessary for initiating infection. However, the strain he used, CN 2726, was passaged many times in guinea pigs and selected for its invasiveness and hence may not be very typical of the majority of toxigenic gangrene strains of *C. perfringens*. Although in every case cited here polyvalent antisera (in other words, containing antibodies to many antigens) were used, Evans had previously established that the protective power of sera in guinea pigs reflected their anti-α but not their anti-θ, -μ, or -κ contents.

Third, active immunity studies were carried out by several groups using different animal species. The best experimental work was done by Boyd *et al* (1972) who extended earlier studies of Owen-Smith. They immunized sheep with a triple antigen containing α-toxoids (all antigenically unrelated) of *C. perfringens, C. novyi*, and *C. septicum*. At intervals up to one year after immunization animals

* It must be remembered that, since gas gangrene is sometimes a mixed infection, oedema could be caused by, for example, *C. novyi* α-toxin and collagen destruction by *C. histolyticum* β-toxin.

were challenged as follows. A piece of battledress, soaked in washed spores of *C. novyi*, was applied to the hind leg of a sheep. A high velocity bullet was fired through the limb of the sheep aimed so as to avoid both the femur and femoral artery. The procedure resulted in deposition of spores deep into muscle and was highly effective in initiating typical gas gangrene. Protected sheep which survived the *C. novyi* challenge were challenged by the same procedure with *C. perfringens* spores in the opposite leg. In all experiments there was a very high degree of protection conferred on vaccinated groups which lasted at least up to one year after vaccination.

Several points from these experiments should be stressed. First, animals surviving challenge at one year had very low α-antitoxin titres but three weeks after challenge these had risen 70-fold. Since control animals died with 72 h it is unlikely that serum antitoxin was raised to protective levels by a secondary response within this period. Thus, low levels of α-antitoxin are protective if present at time of infection. Second, growth and toxin production had occurred because organisms could be cultured from the wound several weeks after challenge and antitoxin titres rose dramatically. This strongly indicates that immunity is antitoxic and not antibacterial. Third, protection was achieved with toxoid preparations made *in vitro*, thereby making it unlikely that there is some as yet unrecognized immunogenic factor produced *in vivo*, at least in respect of the initial lesion. Fourth, in retrospect, the failure to save the lives of some war-wounded patients (Maclennan, 1962) by similar treatment may have been due to the administration of antitoxin too late, the extent and cause of the initial injury, and the possibility that a less typical, highly invasive strain was involved. It is a pity that experiments such as those described by Boyd *et al* (1972) have not been repeated using highly purified toxoids that could easily be prepared today. However, from the existing data one can infer that among the known components of culture filtrates produced *in vitro*, the most likely antigen to be involved is the α-toxin.

What happens when α-toxin produced *in vitro* is injected into animals? Can one reproduce the pathological effects of the disease? Is it responsible for the terminal fatal toxaemia which is so characteristic of gas gangrene? Here, the picture becomes more difficult to analyse and is the most controversial aspect of this subject. Only a few studies will be selected for mention since attempts in the past to reproduce aspects of either the well characterized histological picture of the local lesion or the generalized toxaemia have been carried out with impure preparations. Groups in Sweden, Japan and Ireland have recently contributed a great deal to the purification of *C. perfringens* phospholipase C in particular and bacterial toxins and enzymes in general. They have demonstrated a need to interpret with caution some of the older work with so-called purified α-toxin, particularly of commercial origin, because such preparations are invariably contaminated with other membrane-active components, in particular θ-toxin.

Recently, Sugahara and colleagues showed that highly purified toxin increased the permeability of guinea-pig skin and induced platelet aggregation both *in vitro* and *in vivo*; the latter resulted in production of thrombi and eventual haemostasis. They suggested that the increase in permeability could arise from α-toxin-induced liberation of some unspecified dilator which, from the work of Strandberg and co-workers on rat mast cells, could be histamine. These new observations could help explain the production of oedema and peripheral anoxia, promoting invasion of organisms into adjacent healthy tissue; they could also explain the onset of shock (as discussed in Chapter 6), which characterizes the terminal stages of the disease.

We must be cautious in extrapolating from rodents to man, however. Habermann's experiments using rats, guinea pigs and pigeons showed that the results obtained depended on the choice of animal and route of injection; the importance of these two facts cannot be overstressed to the student in considering this or any other experimental infection. For example, experimental infection is not necessarily fatal in the rat, despite its extreme sensitivity to a-toxin, when administered either intravenously or intramuscularly.

Possibly the most detailed description of experimental intoxication is that of Russian workers (summarized by Ispolatovskaya, 1970) who reproduced the principal features of the disease with semi-purified material. They also suggest that many of the observed changes may not be direct effects of the enzyme but secondary *sequelae* to the release of autodegradative tissue enzymes caused by the degeneration of muscle tissue at the primary site of injection. This view that it is not a-toxin which is responsible for death but some other 'poison', not released or extractable from normal muscle but released from infected muscle, had been advanced earlier to explain the failure of delayed antitoxin therapy and the inability to detect circulating α-toxin in terminal patients.

Finally Strunk and colleagues, in 1967, examined by electron microscopy lesions caused by ferritin-labelled preparations of a-toxin in skeletal muscles of guinea pigs. Ferritin-conjugated toxin appeared in, or was found immediately adjacent to, focal defects of the cytoplasmic membrane. They also observed degeneration of myofilaments. The sarcoplasmic reticulum, mitochondria, and cell nuclei also underwent marked degenerative changes. All of these followed the initial lesions in the cell membrane and occurred independently of the presence of detectable toxin within the cell, and most likely represented changes secondary to the initial lesion in the cell membrane. Similar changes have been described in muscle cells in the context of injury induced by freezing, ischaemia, and in short-term haemorrhagic shock, and are probably the *sequelae* to altered ion-permeability rather than to actual physical disruption of the membrane. Such an interpretation would suggest that damage to mitochondrial structure and oxidative function observed many years ago and periodically revived as possible key events in a-toxin mediated damage are of secondary and not primary significance.

From such observations as these it is difficult to escape the conclusion that the syndrome of fatal human or experimental gas gangrene caused by *C. perfringens* is the integrated sum of all the deranged metabolic events initiated by a-toxin.

Other phospholipases

The foregoing leads naturally to questions as to whether every organism which produces extracellular enzymes of the same or related specificity is pathogenic, or whether every biochemically similar bacterial phospholipase is equally toxic and hence of equal importance as a virulence determinant. The answer to both these questions is no. Table 3 summarized some of the information about the substrate specificity of some bacterial enzymes. Only two of the enzymes are lethal, *C. perfringens* α-toxin and *Corynebacterium ovis* sphingomyelinase D; lethality of staphylococcal β-haemolysin is a controversial point and its role in staphylococcal infections as a cytotoxic agent is discussed in the next chapter.

The lack of correlation between pathogenicity and ability to produce phospholipase C enzymes is not difficult to explain because an organism needs many attributes to be pathogenic, including the ability to adhere, colonize, compete, resist phagocytosis, and so on, in addition to producing potentially toxic factors *in vivo*; without the former the ability to produce toxic enzymes is of little importance. The variation in toxicity is harder to explain. Toxicity is better reflected in the haemolytic activities of these enzyme preparations than in enzymic units. In particular it is possible to show that the rate of haemolysis is dependent upon red-cell concentration. An 'apparent Km' value for haemolysin can therefore be obtained, reflecting the affinity of the enzyme for its substrate *in situ*; the value for *C. perfringens* α-toxin is four times greater than for *C. bifermentans* phospholipase C. Thus toxicity, judged by lethal capacity or haemolytic capacity, is not inherent in phospholipases of a particular biochemical type, nor is susceptibility to this kind of phospholipase inherent in a cell containing lecithin. The toxicity is the resultant of the rate of action of the enzyme, which is dependent primarily on the relationship between the enzyme and the substrate *in situ* in the cell and, presumably, the rate of cell repair.

It is important to stress that hydrolysis of the phospholipids in a cell does not necessarily lead to cell disintegration. For example, staphylococcal β-haemolysin, which probably has the narrowest substrate specificity, is a hot–cold haemolysin, lysis of erythrocytes occurring only on cooling after incubation at 37°C. The phenomenon, though of doubtful significance *in vivo*, has attracted attention and generated speculation about its mechanism. Perhaps the most likely explanation is that, when cooled below their phase-transition temperature, the remaining phospholipids undergo quasi-crystalline formation, thereby generating intra-membranous stresses incompatible with structural integrity.

C. perfringens α-toxin is another example of a hot–cold haemolysin. The term is clearly a misnomer because lysis is a secondary effect on cells after exposure to phospholipase activity. To describe a cell as being susceptible to hot–cold haemolysis is more accurate than describing an enzyme as a hot–cold haemolysin. *C. ovis* spingomyelinase D does not cause lysis of erythrocytes, despite the effective removal of choline from spingomyelin, easily demonstrated by failure of staphylococcal sphingomyelinase C and *C. perfringens* phospholipase C to cause lysis after treatment with sphingomyelinase D.

Thiol-activated cytolysins

These proteins (Table 4) have been called oxygen-labile haemolysins because they are reversibly inactivated on standing in air and their most studied property is their ability to lyse red cells. The modern view is that SH-activation as such is necessary for the expression of haemolytic activity and that they are active towards a variety of cell types. In fact, it is the recognition of what these substances do to host defence cells when presented in sub-lethal doses that has increased interest in this group of proteins as factors of potential but as yet unproven relevance in microbial pathogenicity. Thiol-activated cytolysins share the following properties: they are cross-neutralized by hyperimmune sera, lyse a wide range of species of erythocyte, exhibit similar pH and temperature optima for cytolytic activity, are lethal and cardiotoxic, and lose activity on incubation with erythrocyte ghosts. Finally, they are inactivated irreversibly by small amounts of cholesterol; it is for this reason that we are considering these substances here, because the evidence is that interaction with cholesterol is the key primary event in their interaction with susceptible membranes which leads to the impairment of the latter.

Activation; structural relatedness Until recently there was no evidence to substantiate an S–S reduction step by thiol compounds as the mechanism of SH activation. However, amino acid analysis of cereolysin has recently revealed the presence of two half cystine residues/molecule, thereby providing the possible basis for reductive activation. The amino acid compositions of at least three of these haemolysins differ widely, which is remarkable in view of the high degree of immunological similarity that exists between them. The latter feature implies similarity of secondary and tertiary structures. On the basis of serological tests, Alouf has ascribed at least two functionally distinct regions to these proteins, the 'f' (fixation) and 'l' (lytic) sites, regarded as important in a speculative mechanism he has put forward to explain their mode of haemolytic action (see below).

Inhibition by cholesterol Haemolysis by thiol-activated cytolysins is inhibited irreversibly by cholesterol and stereospecifically related sterols; the common structural features necessary for inhibition are the presence of an OH group in the β-configuration on C_3 and an iso-octyl side chain on C_{17} (Fig. 2). Only cells containing cholesterol in their plasma membranes (most mammalian cells) are susceptible, whereas those lacking in cholesterol (bacterial protoplasts, certain mycoplasmas, for example) are insusceptible to SH-activated cytolysins. Additional evidence that cholesterol-containing liposomes inactivate, whereas cholesterol-lacking liposomes do not inactivate, SH-activated cytolysins, strongly argues in favour of cholesterol being the primary binding site of these cytolysins.

Table 4 *SH-activated cytolysins*

Species	Name(s)	Properties summarized in two source references (a) and (b)
streptococci, groups A, B, C and G	streptolysin O	Molecular weights, isoelectric points, amino acid compositions, lethality, comparative
Streptococcus pneumoniae	pneumolysin	susceptibilities of erythrocytes of different species,
Clostridium tetani	tetanolysin	cholesterol-SH-cytolysin
C. perfringens	perfringolysin (θ-toxin)	stoichiometry.
C. septicum	septicolysin (δ-toxin)	These are not reproduced
C. histolyticum	histolyticolysin (ε-toxin)	here since for some there are
C. oedematiens type A	oedematolysin (δ-toxin)	wide variations in the experi-
C. bifermentans	bifermentolysin	mental data.
C. chauvoei	chauveolysin (δ-toxin)	
C. sordelli	sordelliolysin	
C. caproicum	caproiciolysin	
C. botulinum	botulinolysin	
Bacillus cereus	cereolysin	
B. thuringiensis	thuringiolysin 0	
B. alvei	alveolysin	
B. laterosporus	laterosporolysin	
Listeria monocytogenes	listeriolysin	

Information compiled from (a) C. J. Smyth and J. L. Duncan (1978) in *Bacterial Toxins and Cell Membranes* p. 129, ed. by J. Jeljaszewicz and T. Wadström (Academic Press) and (b) A. W. Bernheimer (1976) in *Mechanisms in Bacterial Toxinology* p. 85. ed. by A. W. Bernheimer (Wiley).

Mechanism of action Smyth and Duncan describe current ideas, and the experimental evidence on which they are based, in Jeljaszewicz and Wadström (1978). Hence, only a brief summary will be given here. Thiol-activated cytolysin binds to cholesterol, a step which is temperature independent. At 0°C, the formation of toxin-cholesterol complexes does not induce morphological changes, as judged by electron microscope studies, or weakening of the membrane as judged by osmotic fragility measurements. At this stage the toxin may be neutralized by antitoxin but not by cholesterol. On warming to 37°C a series of structures varying from arcs and c-shapes to closed rings become visible. These are interpreted as aggregations of toxin-cholesterol complexes which were originally dispersed throughout the membrane, or of sequestration of cholesterol by ring-like aggregates of toxin.

The net result, predictable by either interpretation, is the effective withdrawal of cholesterol from general distribution throughout the membrane. This would alter profoundly the physical and functional integrity of the membrane, leading to permeability changes. These ring structures of presumptive toxin-cholesterol complexes may peel off, thus physically removing cholesterol from, and not just redistributing it, within the membrane. The arc/ring structures have been shown by freeze-etching to be pits and not trans-membranous holes. Thus leakage from, and the eventual lysis of cells is to be seen as a sequel to the induction of 'functional holes', which arise from structural reorientation and weakening of the membrane, rather than the drilling of 'physical holes'.

Alouf has postulated two distinct sites on the streptolysin-O molecule—*f*, which fixes or binds to cholesterol, and *l*, which is involved in triggering lysis—based on antibody-mediated blocking of haemolysis. Alouf's model is not inconsistent with that of Smyth and Duncan. There is no problem with *f*. However, the need to postulate an active function for *l* in causing complex aggregate-formation with cholesterol is uncertain since above the phase-transition temperature lateral diffusion could account for this. The blocking effects of anti-*l* antibody could be due to steric hindrance as much as neutralization of some secondary activity of the protein.

Role in disease This is a more difficult question. Streptolysin-O is lethal for rabbits, mice, rats and guinea pigs due to cardiotoxic rather than haemolytic effects, but there is no evidence that in tetanus, or gas gangrene, for example or in streptococcal infections such factors play any significant role in disease. The most studied member of this group of proteins is streptolysin-O. It is definitely produced in human infections; a rise in anti-streptolysin-O antibody titre is a diagnostic test for streptococcal infection.

In view of the known cardiotoxicity of these proteins, the action of streptolysin-O on heart muscle has been put forward as an alternative explanation of the cause of rheumatic fever; this 'direct action' view is in contrast to the widely accepted autoimmune mechanism in which cardiac muscle is damaged by hypersensitivity mechanisms arising from cross-reactions between streptococcal and heart antigens. However, apart from their much studied haemolytic property, thiol-activated cytolysins are known to interact with a variety of leucocytes, in particular those involved in host defence mechanisms; the data on this aspect have been summarized in Jeljaszewicz and Wadström (1978). Streptolysin-O markedly inhibits the chemotactic and random movement of human neutrophils, but not monocytes. This effect seems to be on the locomotor and not the orientating mechanism and is not immunologically mediated. Streptolysin-O also induces rapid degranulation of rabbit leucocytes, inhibits the phytohaemagglutinin-induced transformation of lymphocytes, and alters the functional integrity of human fibroblast membranes; *C. perfringens θ*-toxin causes the release of histamine from platelets and alters vascular permeability.

It is evident from the properties displayed by this group of bacterial cytolysins that they are capable of playing a role in infection. However, one must not forget that *there is no positive evidence at present to implicate them in disease* and further attempts to do so should be concentrated on searching at the sub-lethal level for possible effects *in vivo* which may contribute to the overall picture of bacterial pathogenicity.

Toxins with a surfactant mechanism

This section is included to indicate the possibility of another type of mechanism whereby bacterial products could damage cell membranes—that is, by a detergent-like effect: two products are known, staphylococcal *δ*-toxin and subtilysin produced by *Bacillus subtilis*. The case for considering *δ*-toxin as a determinant of staphylococcal pathogenicity is argued in the next chapter, while there is none for subtilysin, since *B. subtilis* is not normally a pathogen.

Subtilysin consists of a heptapeptide linked to a long-chain fatty acid. Its properties are similar to those of staphylococcal *δ*-toxin and melittin, the principal cytolysin of bee venom. Delta-toxin is a heat stable peptide of molecular weight 5000 daltons, is now accepted as antigenic, has a high proportion (30–40 per cent) of hydrophobic amino acids, and causes lesions in membranes strikingly similar to those caused by melittin and the detergent Triton X-100, although the lesions produced by the toxins are initially smaller than those of Triton X-100. Delta toxin is thought to be a surfactant because it is inhibited by phospholipids and dilute normal serum, is soluble in chloroform/methanol (2 : 1 by vol), has a low specific haemolytic activity, lyses a wide range of cell types, and dissolves membranes rather like sodium deoxycholate.

For a summary of this chapter see the end of Chapter 4 (page 58).

References

BOYD, N. A., THOMSON, R. O. & WALKER, P. D. (1972). 'The prevention of experimental *Clostridium novyi* and *C. perfringens* gas gangrene in high-velocity missile wounds by active immunization.' *J. Med. Microbiol.* 5: 467.

ISPOLATOVSKAYA, M. V. (1971). 'Type A *Clostridium perfringens* toxin.' In: *Microbial Toxins* Vol. IIA, p. 109. Edited by S. Kadis, T. C. Montie and S. J. Ajl. Academic Press.

JELJASZEWICZ, J. & WADSTRÖM, T. Eds. (1978). *Bacterial toxins and cell membranes.* Academic Press.

MACLENNAN, J. D. (1962). 'The histotoxic clostridial infections of man.' *Bact. Rev.* 26: 177.

STRUNK, S. W., SMITH, C. W. & BLUMBERG, J. M. (1967). 'Ultrastructural studies on the lesion produced in skeletal muscle fibres by crude type A *Clostridium perfringens* toxin and its purified alpha fraction.' *Am. J. Path. 50*: 89.

WISEMAN, G. M. (1975). 'The haemolysins of *Staphylococcus aureus*.' *Bact. Rev. 39*: 317.

4 Membrane-damaging toxins; primary event not known

Staphylococcal toxins

Although we mentioned two staphylococcal toxins (β and δ) in Chapter 3 we have delayed discussion on the possible pathogenic significance of these until this chapter, which includes three other staphylococcal toxins, α, γ, and leucocidin. There are similarities between the status of staphylococcal α-toxin and that of *C. perfringens* α-toxin in that each has been regarded by many to be a very (and by some the most) important toxin elaborated by these respective pathogens. Evidence for the importance of *C. perfringens* α-toxin was outlined in Chapter 3, but similar evidence concerning the relevance of staphylococcal α-toxin in disease production is more difficult to adduce.

Staphylococci are ubiquitous and responsible for a large range of clinically different diseases which range from the relatively harmless skin pimple through abscesses, impetigo, food-poisoning, osteomyelitis, mastitis, primary pneumonia, staphylococcal scalded skin syndrome (SSSS), to fatal septicaemias.

It was the accidental case of fatal septicaemia involving 21 children in 1928 at Bundaberg in Australia that originally focused attention on the existence of lethal factors produced by staphylococci. They were inoculated with a diphtheria toxin-antitoxin preparation and within 48 h twelve of the children were dead. *Staphylococcus aureus* was isolated from the 'immunizing' preparation, which was also shown to be haemolytic and lethal for rabbits. The terminal symptoms of the children suggested that they died from the effects of a haemolytic toxin. This focused attention on four staphylococcal haemolysins α, β, γ, δ, together with a possible fifth, ε, whose separate existence is still disputed. There is little doubt that in such fatal septicaemias—which are now rare among staphylococcal infections—that toxins are important, and that α-toxin in particular is the agent of death. In the cases of food poisoning and SSSS the toxins responsible are well known, though not their modes of action, and these will be discussed in the next chapter.

Staphylococcal α-toxin Because of the now well-recognized synergistic effects of certain combinations of staphylococcal toxins observable at the cytotoxic level, the older literature on cell susceptibility to α-toxin must be interpreted with caution. Extensive studies of membrane and lipid interactions have been recently carried out with highly purified toxin (molecular weight 26–39 000 daltons: four forms by isoelectric focusing). Rabbit erythrocytes are far more susceptible to haemolysis by α-toxin than those of other species; for example, human erythrocytes are approximately 1 000 times less sensitive. Despite this, morphological studies using high concentrations of toxin reveal the formation of ring-like structures of α-toxin on a variety of cellular membranes. These can also be induced in aqueous dispersions of individual lipids; they also penetrate monolayers of different lipids to differing degrees.

Freeze-etching studies reveal that α-toxin causes marked changes in the hydrophobic fracture plane of rabbit erythrocyte membranes, superficially resembling those associated with the thiol-activated lysins discussed in Chapter 3; however, no one specific lipid has been identified as the target of primary interaction. From such studies Freer and Arbuthnott interpreted staphylococcal α-toxin to be a 'surface active' factor, but Wiseman and colleagues disagree. In their view α-toxin is activated by membrane enzymes and causes lysis by proteolytic action on membrane proteins, but Freer and colleagues were unable to confirm this. In support, Wiseman points out that Cassidy and colleagues showed that liposomes prepared from lipids extracted from rabbit and human erythrocytes were equally susceptible to lysis by α-toxin despite the enormous difference in susceptibility of the respective cells. In Wiseman's model, the ring-like structures would be interpreted as the orientation of the initially adsorbed toxin to render it susceptible to activation. Thus, there is disagreement about the mechanism of lytic action of α-toxin which only further experimentation will clarify.

Thelestam and co-workers have shown that α-toxin induces smaller functional pores in human diploid lung fibroblasts (HDLF) than in HeLa cells. Such differences between cells, together with the fact that washed membranes bind 12–14 times as much toxin as do whole cells, require that one extrapolates from such studies to situations *in vivo* only with great caution.

From the foregoing only one thing is clear: α-toxin interacts with membranes. At present we cannot predict the spectrum of cell susceptibility or explain its pharmacological effects on smooth muscle, or its dermonecrotic, haemolytic, and lethal effects.

Staphylococcal γ-toxin This is a complex toxin consisting of two proteins (I and II, molecular weights 29 000 and 26 000 daltons respectively), each of which is inactive on its own but which together act synergistically. γ-toxin is lytic to rabbit, but much less so to sheep and human erythrocytes. Its haemolytic action is inhibited by several lipids, but there is no evidence for degradation of such compounds or of a thiol-activated cytolysin/cholesterol type of interaction. Only studies by Fackrell and Wiseman, who killed guinea pigs by intracardial injection, constitute evidence for whole-animal toxicity; injection of rabbits (subcutaneously), mice (intraperitoneally or intravenously), or guinea pigs (subcutaneously) with purified γ-toxin had no effect. Thelestam and co-workers failed to show release of ^{3}H-uridine by γ-toxin from HDLF and HeLa cells in their test system, but Fackrell and Wiseman claim that it damages leucocytes.

Staphylococcal leucocidin (Panton-Valentine or PV leucocidin) Even though there may be doubts about the role of PV-leucocidin as a determinant of staphylococcal pathogenicity, the leucocidin complex recognized by Panton and Valentine in 1932 has attracted the attention of those searching for protective staphylococcal antigens. The admirable studies of Woodin serve as a model for those who would seek to understand the molecular interactions of other synergistic complex toxins.

PV-leucocidin shows a remarkable specificity for the polymorphonuclear neutrophils and macrophages of man and rabbit. Until very recently no other biological activity was attributed to this toxin, but Ward and co-workers have recently shown that purified leucocidin (purified and crystallyzed by Woodin) evokes a dermonecrotic response in rabbits: as yet the cellular basis of this reaction has not been elucidated.

The toxin consists of two components, F (fast) and S (slow), so designated because of their relative rates of migration on carboxymethyl cellulose. The effect of the toxin on leucocytes is to cause a change in cation permeability, in particular an efflux of K^+ and an influx of Ca^{2+}; phosphate, nucleotides, sugars, and cytoplasmic proteins are not released from the leucocidin-treated cell. However, treatment of polymorphonuclear neutrophils causes discharge of protein into the medium from the characteristic degradative granules of these cells. In addition, certain membrane enzymes are activated—acyl phosphatases, which may be components of the potassium pump in the leucocyte, and adenylate cyclase. Woodin suggested that the changes in the leucocidin-treated cell are all secondary *sequelae* to the primary event, which is altered cation permeability; if Ca^{2+} was removed from the external medium, then secondary effects such as degranulation did not occur.

Current ideas are that introduction of Ca^{2+} into the cytoplasmic compartment of many cells by physiological means (for example, by hormonal stimuli) or by non-physiological means (for example, by ionophores, or energy-depletion of cells) has several *sequelae*. These include the opening of a K^+ gate, allowing efflux of K^+ into the external medium, and the activation of 'Ca^{2+}-activated regulator protein', which controls several membrane-bound enzyme systems and secretory activities of specialized cells. It is possible to interpret most of Woodin's findings within this new framework.

How then does leucocidin bring about these primary membrane changes? Incubation of radio-labelled F and S components with cells shows that only a small and fairly constant amount of the radioactivity is bound to the cells and the leucocidin in solution becomes inactivated. These results strongly suggest that the site of action is the membrane.

Further experiments with leucocidin involving both cell membranes and phospholipids at different ionic strengths reveal that the interaction is extremely complex resulting in polymerization as well as inactivation of the leucocidin. At low ionic strength in the presence of aqueous suspensions of phosphatidyl serine, di- and triphosphoinositides and phosphatidyl choline, but not other phospholipids, F is converted to a polymeric form. The process is reversed at high ionic strength and by low concentration of Ca^{2+}. F is presumed to react with the fatty acid side-chains of the micelle constituents because 'free' polar head groups do not inhibit polymerization with phosphoglycerides, and diglycerides induce polymerization. S component is not polymerized by phospholipids (although it is by membranes at low ionic strength), and adsorbs to micelles by interacting with F after its adsorption and modification by phospholipids. These and other observations lead to the conclusion that F interacts first with membranes, in particular with the hydrophobic interior of membranes, which induces a conformational state in F capable of adsorbing S component.

The next step is postulated from two observations. First, the only phospholipid in leucocyte membranes to inactivate leucocidin is triphosphoinositide. Second, component S is inactivated at physiological and not at low ionic strength, suggesting an interaction with the hydrophilic regions of phospholipids. No stable complexes or covalent interactions occur. As yet the simultaneous inactivation of F and S has not been demonstrated in aqueous dispersions containing only triphosphoinositide and leucocidin. If, as is assumed by Woodin, the inactivation of leucocidin by triphosphoinositide is simultaneous or synonymous with the mechanism responsible for controlling K^+ permeability, then the stereospecific configurations assumed by F and S in the membrane must be such that the hydrophobic and hydrophilic regions of the membrane are equally accessible to F and S, creating a functional pore. Efflux of K^+ and influx of Ca^{2+} through this 'pore region' would increase the ionic strength of the region and result in the deformation of the F-phospholipid complex (as described above) and subsequent release and dissociation of the S–F complex into two inactive proteins (adsorbed F, though depolymerized, is not reactivated at high ionic strength). Woodin has also suggested that interaction of F and S causes a conformational change in the head group of triphosphoinositide, which is reversed after desorption at the expense of cellular ATP, allowing the cycle of events to be repeated with fresh leucocidin molecules.

There is sufficient triphophoinositide in leucocyte membranes to account for the observations, but presence of triphosphoinositide cannot be the whole story, since this is known to be present in cells not susceptible to the effect of leucocidin. The specificity of the interaction between leucocidin and susceptible cells, therefore, must reflect the presence of another primary receptor or the accessibility of triphosphoinositide in leucocytes to the F and S components of leucocidin.

Role of staphylococcal toxins in infection This is not an easy subject on which to say much that is original or to summarize concisely what has already been said. Much contemporary research concerns staphylococcal pathogenicity and not the pathogenesis of staphylococcal infections. The former relates to the potential of staphylococci to cause disease and is often studied *in vitro* or by injecting large numbers of organisms into mice or rabbits. Pathogenesis concerns the mechanisms of disease production *in vivo*. This has proved very difficult to analyse and may or may not involve staphylococcal toxins.

The elucidation of the factors which convert the ubiquitous staphylococcal saprophyte (or harmless commensal) to a pathogen constitutes one of the important extant challenges in bacterial pathogenicity, mainly because no one has yet developed a really suitable model for studying the pathogenesis of the classical local lesion, the abscess, a brief description of which follows.

The presence of bacteria in some local site initiates an inflammatory response; that is, recruitment to the site of polymorphonuclear cells (white phagocytic cells which possess granules containing degradative enzymes capable of destroying microbes if these are ingested, or damaging host tissues if released extracellularly), accompanied by exudation of plasma constituents. If, during the initial inflammatory response, bacteria are not ingested and destroyed, more phagocytes and fluid accumulate. When fully developed such a lesion will have a central necrotic core, filled with dead cells and bacteria, which is walled off from surrounding tissue by a deposition of fibrin, entrapped in which are viable cocci and phagocytic cells. The centre may continue to liquefy, generating tension and increasing local pain and tenderness; it may burst, drain and heal without assistance. This kind of infection usually remains localized and rarely leads to gross systemic effects. Small laboratory animals have never been successfully used to produce this type of lesion at will, particularly on the skin. Parenteral injection of virulent staphylococci will either kill the animal (probably due to α-toxin production) or cause abscess-formation in a variety of internal organs. The best experimental animal is perhaps the human, although even here there are problems.

There is no absolute correlation between virulence (as determined by clinical origin or by lethality for rabbits or mice) and the ability to produce toxins *in vitro*. Table 5 shows that staphylococci produce a wide range of extracellular products, of which only coagulase is considered to correlate with, if not be a determinant of, virulence. Gladstone and Glencross, in 1960, showed that some coagulase-positive strains from human sources which were uniformly haemolysin-negative on blood

Table 5 Extracellular toxins and other products produced by staphylococci

	Physico-chemical data*			
		Number of		
		electro-	pI	
	Molecular	phoretic	main	Main biological
Product	weight	forms	form	properties
α-haemolysin	29–36 000	4	8.5	lethal, dermonecrotic, haemolytic (rabbit rbc's most sensitive) spastic paralysis smooth muscle
β-haemolysin	30 000	2	9.4	lethal (?) hot-cold haemolysin, (sensitivity of rbc: sheep human, rabbit)
γ-haemolysin factor I	29 000	1	9.8	synergistic mixture,
γ-haemolysin factor II	26 000		9.9	lethal, haemolytic
δ-haemolysin	103 000 (sub-unit 5 000)	2	9.5	lethal (?), haemolytic surfactant
leucocidin F	32 000	1	9.0	synergistic mixture,
leucocidin S	38 000			toxic to human and rabbit PMNs and macrophages, dermonecrotic
exfoliatin	25 000	2	7.0	intra-epidermal cleavage
enterotoxin A	27 800	4	7.3	
enterotoxin B	28 366	4	8.6	
enterotoxin C_1	34 100	3	8.6	
enterotoxin C_2	34 000	3–8	7.0	
enterotoxin E	29 600		7.0	

Other factors include neuraminidase, hyaluronidase, lipase, DNAse, staphylokinase (activates plasminogen, dissolves clots), staphylocoagulase (activates prothrombin and fibrinogen but not other clotting factors). In addition there are cell-bound factors which include clumping factor (coagulase) involved in para-coagulation of fibrinogen. Only coagulase activity seems to be correlated with a high frequency with virulence.

* Physico-chemical data reproduced with permission from McCartney A. C. and Arbuthnott J. P. (1978). In *Bacterial toxins and cell membranes*. Ed. by J. Jeljaszewicz and T. Wadström, Academic Press.

agar plates all produced α-haemolysin when grown in 'Cellophane' sacs implanted in the rabbit. In fact, there is evidence that α, β and γ haemolysins and leucocidin are produced *in vivo* during natural and experimental infections. This is based on the presence of antibodies to these haemolysins in subjects undergoing staphylococcal infection and the extraction of α-haemolysin from peritoneal abscesses in mice, or in mammary gland homogenates from lactating mice inoculated with some (but not all) strains of staphylococci. Thus, some of the toxins are produced *in vivo*. Therefore, we can meaningfully ask two crucial questions. Can we reproduce the principal features of disease, in particular the local lesion, by injecting toxin, or prevent the development of the lesion by prophylactic antitoxin therapy?

The study of the role of toxins in the causation, and antitoxin in the prevention, of staphylococcal disease in the human reached its peak in the pre-antibiotic era and was never satisfactorily resolved. Interest in these aspects declined as the therapeutic success of antibiotics rose. However, interest in mechanisms of staphylococcal pathogenicity has been rekindled in this era of antibiotic resistance, and the availability of highly purified toxin preparations is itself a good reason for reworking some of the older ground.

This rather diffuse area has been reviewed by Elek (1959) and more recently by Wiseman (1975) with little evidence of substantial progress in the intervening period. The first point to make is that pyogenic staphylococcal infections do not confer immunity to the patient after recovery. Therefore, the role of toxins in establishing localized lesions is exceedingly difficult to analyse by selective administration of antitoxin or pre-immunization with toxoids. From the pre-pencillin era, during which antitoxic therapy was practised, no clear consensus emerged about the relative importance of the corresponding antigens in disease production. In 1959, Elek wrote 'The protection afforded by alpha antitoxin, whether acquired by active or passive immunization, has been described repeatedly and at length by a small group of workers. *Neither repetition nor eloquence renders the theme more convincing.* The experimental work is based mainly on rabbits and mice, two species with high susceptibility to the lethal effect of alpha toxin. The free toxin in the challenging dose of a whole culture overshadows the picture in such experiments, and it is not surprising that animals with high antitoxin levels in their blood survive. Even the most sanguine protagonists of the importance of antitoxin have been forced to admit, however, that the development of local metastatic lesions is not prevented by antitoxin, and generally all that may be shown is slightly longer survival of immunized animals. It was held that the origin of the antitoxin was immaterial; as long as it was present in sufficiently high amount in the circulating blood, both active immunization by toxoid and passive serum treatment was said to produce immunity in rabbits'. This position has changed little in the intervening 20 years.

In the case of mastitis the picture changes somewhat. The enormous economic importance of this disease in the dairying industry has resulted in considerable research on this topic in the bovine, but this is very expensive and the gestation and lactation periods slow down progress in *in vivo* studies; small laboratory animals models are therefore very important, and for some aspects of mastitis apparently relevant.

Anderson inoculated the mammary glands of lactating mice with two strains of staphylococci isolated from acute and chronic clinical cases of bovine mastitis. Strain BB was a 'high virulence' strain causing a gangrenous type of mastitis (characterized by a complete absence of healthy polymorphonuclear neutrophils

(PMNs)), and sometimes death, whereas strain Mexi was most frequently associated with a chronic mastitis which only sometimes became acute. The apparent key difference when these two strains were inoculated into mice was their ability to survive intraphagocytic digestion in the mammary gland. Strain BB was more efficient in this respect and outpaced the rate at which additional host defence mechanisms could be mounted, or destroyed them. Strong evidence for a role for α-toxin was adduced: it could be extracted from homogenates of infected glands, was always present when animals died, and histopathological examination revealed an absence of healthy PMN cells and presence of extracellular bacteria. Apart from the presence of bacterial cells, the pathology could be reproduced by injection of sterile toxin preparations known to contain α-toxin. The effect on leucocytes could scarcely be due to PV-leucocidin as it is highly specific for human and rabbit leucocytes. Repetition of these key experiments with highly purified material and attempts to neutralize the effects with appropriate antisera could, in principle, answer absolutely the question about the role that α-toxin (or any other staphylococcal factor) plays in this system.

Adlam and colleagues studied a naturally occurring staphylococcal mastitis in rabbits and tested some postulates about the pathogenic roles of various factors using *purified* preparations. The naturally occurring disease in lactating rabbits is characterized by abscess-formation from which animals recover slowly without development of immunity to subsequent infection. Rabbits cannot be protected using a vaccine comprising the causative organism and its formalin-treated products (produced *in vitro*). The disease can be reproduced in the laboratory by injecting the mammary gland or by allowing lactating does to suckle litters infected intranasally with the causative organism.

Under these conditions, two forms of disease, similar to that described by Anderson in mice, occurred, reflecting the field situation in cattle. These were a local abscess, non-lethal disease and 'blue breast', characterized by oedematous haemorrhagic mammary tissue and further damage spreading to sites distant from the initial site of infection and rapid death; such distal sites were often sterile. Vaccination with crude vaccine did not prevent 'blue breast' but did convert it to the local abscess-type of disease. Only α-toxoid was effective in preventing 'blue breast' when two strains (one of which was BB, the gangrenous bovine strain used by Anderson) were used to challenge the immunized group. This accords with work done by Derbyshire and Smith, who converted gangrenous mastitis in goats to the more chronic type by immunization with a crude vaccine which induced high levels of α-antitoxin. However, in further experiments Adlam and colleagues (personal communication) immunized animals with purified PV-leucocidin or γ-toxin, either alone or in combination with α-toxin. No protection was afforded against challenge with the strain of staphylococci isolated from naturally occurring mastitis in rabbits: indeed, some animals contracted 'blue breast' in spite of circulating antibodies to α-toxin. They concluded that, in a proportion of does challenged by the natural rabbit strain, 'blue breast' may also be caused by an, as yet, unidentified toxin.

The importance of healthy PMNs in maintaining a balance between chronic and gangrenous mastitis has been demonstrated by Schalin and co-workers who converted a chronic type to a gangrenous type of disease by using anti-PMN sera. Thus the role of α-toxin may be leucocidal, enabling rapid multiplication of organisms and elaboration of lethal levels of α-toxin. Alpha-antitoxin, therefore, may prevent the destruction of the cells which results in abscess formation.

Promise for the future lies in the recognition of a type of synergism—different from that observed between components of a single complex toxin—between two separate toxic entities. Thelestam and co-workers have shown that sublytic amounts of δ-toxin cause release of cell constituents without lysis. Perhaps more important is the fact that only 0.01 haemolytic units of α-toxin will cause lysis of cells in the presence of 0.004 units of δ-toxin. This synergistic interaction could be the way in which staphylococcal toxins, which rarely exert their lethal effects in the majority of infections, exercise important cytolytic effects. Of less obvious significance is the fact that δ-toxin is a poor antigen; its antigenicity was controversial until very recently. If δ-toxin were to prove of crucial importance as a cytolytic potentiator, then this could also partly explain why natural acquired immunity is either non-existent or sufficiently low as to be easily overcome.

Streptococcal toxins

It has become customary for reviewers to include, in sections on membrane-damaging toxins, a statement about streptococcal toxins. Like staphylococci, β-haemolytic streptococci produce a range of extracellular toxins and enzymes: these include streptolysin-O, streptolysin-S, erythrogenic toxins (see Chapter 5), various nucleases, NAD-glychoydrolase, streptokinase (fibrinolysin), proteinase, and hyaluronidase. A variety of human infections (including sore throats, scarlet fever, rheumatic fever, and glomerulo-nephritis) are caused by so-called β-haemolytic streptococci, organisms characterized by production of a clear zone of haemolysis on fresh blood agar.

Most of the important human pathogens are β-haemolytic and can be classified into Lancefield groups A, B, C, and so on, based on the nature of the polysaccharide present on the surface of the organism; most human pathogens are group A. Within these broad groupings, they can be further subdivided according to surface protein antigens M, T, or R; M protein is of considerable importance as a virulence factor because it inhibits phagocytosis. The cell-wall peptidoglycan (as in staphylococci) is a pyrogen and can also induce the local Schwartzman reaction (see Chapter 6).

In contrast to some of the cell-wall constituents, there is no good evidence to implicate any known streptococcal extracellular toxin or other factor in pathogenicity. Two cytolytic factors are known: the much studied streptolysin-O, a thiol-activated cytolysin referred to in the previous chapter, and streptolysin-S.

Streptolysin-S is responsible for the β-zone of haemolysis surrounding streptococcal colonies on blood agar, but it is not known whether the toxin is produced *in vivo* because it is not antigenic and so no antibodies can be detected in convalescent sera. This lysin has not been isolated in a purified form, but it is thought to be a peptide comprising 28 amino acids. It may be associated with a carrier molecule, the nature of which can vary. Another 'intracellular' lysin exists with similar, though not identical, properties. Streptolysin-S causes lysis of erythrocytes by a mechanism as yet not defined, but quite different from that described above for streptolysin-O, and which probably involves several phospholipids. Phosphatidyl-choline, -ethanolamine and phosphatidic acid inhibit streptolysin-S, and pretreatment of cells with phospholipase C diminishes binding of the toxin, suggesting a receptor-binding (substrate?) role for membrane-phospholipids in streptolysin-S action.

Streptolysin-S is toxic to leucocytes, but the nature of the carrier molecule determines the rate at which cells degranulate and die; in sub-toxic doses phagocytosis is inhibited. It also lyses blood platelets and is toxic to several established cell lines. Streptolysin-S is lethal for mice, several organs (kidney, lung, heart, vascular beds) being affected, but its role in the pathogenesis of streptococcal infections is not clear. However, its properties suggest that a possible pathogenic role for this substance cannot be ruled out.

Finally, Okamoto and co-workers over many years have tried to identify the anti-tumour principle of streptococci; it may or may not be streptolysin-S.

Other membrane-damaging toxins

Doubtless further work will reveal that other bacterial toxins are membrane-active. For example, the α-toxin of *Clostridium novyi* which produces such massive oedema, α-toxins of *C. septicum* and *C. histolyticum*, and anthrax toxin which, according to one view, induces secondary shock by altering vascular permeability may, with others, be described in future in this, rather than the next, chapter.

Summary of Chapters 3 and 4

Membrane-damaging toxins form a large, expanding, heterogeneous group comprising substances which may modify phospholipids, sequester cholesterol, possess detergent-like properties, and others whose primary mode of action cannot yet be specified.

Cell lysis is not an automatic sequel to toxin-membrane interaction; increased membrane permeability or fragility at lower temperatures may result.

As exemplified by the phospholipases, definition of the biochemical mode of action of one toxin does not *a priori* mean that all substances with the same or similar mode of action will be equally toxic or relevant in pathogenicity.

The possible mode of action of staphylococcal leucocidin is currently better understood than any other synergistic toxin complex.

The problems of assigning definitive roles to specific toxins of putative significance in the pathogenesis of acute lethal and localized non-lethal infection caused by organisms which produce a multiplicity of potentially important extracellular factors, is exemplified by the discussion of *C. perfringens* α-toxin and staphylococcal toxins.

References

ADLAM, C., WARD, P. D., MCCARTNEY, A. C., ARBUTHNOTT, J. P., & THORLEY, C. M. (1977). 'Effect of immunization with highly purified α- and β-toxins on staphylococcal mastitis in rabbits.' *Inf. and Imm.* 17: 250.

ELEK, S. D. (1959). *Staphylococcus pyogenes and its relation to disease.* Churchill Livingstone, Edinburgh.

WISEMAN, G. M. (1975). 'The haemolysins of *Staphylococcus aureus.*' *Bact. Rev. 39*: 317.

WOODIN, A. M. (1970). 'Staphylococcal leucocidin.' In: *Microbial Toxins* Vol III p. 327. Edited by T. C. Montie, S. Kadis, and S. J. Ajl. Academic Press.

5 Toxins of known importance in the genesis of specific lesions; mode of action not known

In this section we shall consider a number of toxins for which there is, as yet, little information on their biochemical modes of action but weighty, and in some cases unequivocal, evidence for their role in the genesis of specific lesions or disease syndromes.

Anthrax toxin

Anthrax occurs in two forms. The first is the localized cutaneous infection which is readily treated by antibiotics and which occurs in man, swine, rabbits, and horses. It occurs rarely in humans, mainly among veterinarians, meat workers and in woollen mills—hence the name 'wool-sorters' disease'. The second or septicaemic form may develop from untreated cutaneous infection or by primary infection *via* the respiratory and gastro-intestinal routes or infection of wounds.

Generalized anthrax is nearly always fatal. Herbivores are the usual victims, with cattle, sheep, horses and goats, in that order, being most susceptible. Mice and guinea pigs are the most susceptible laboratory animals, but monkeys have also been used as models for human infections. The organism is highly invasive, spreading throughout the body from the initial portal of entry, producing a characteristic massive terminal bacteraemia. In certain parts of the world it is of sufficient economic importance to warrant vaccination of animals at risk and this can be done with live attenuated strains.

Before the 1950s, no toxin had been recognized as a possible cause of death by this highly invasive pathogen. Various suggestions had been put forward, including hyperglycaemia, Ca^{2+} imbalance, damage to the central nervous system, and anoxia resulting from mechanical blockage of capillaries by massive terminal bacteraemia. Instead, from the early 1900s to late 1940s, observations had accumulated on the aggressin-activity of this organism, that is, its ability to counteract possible host defence mechanisms, in particular interference with phagocytic activity and anthracidal activity of tissue fluids. Immunity to the disease could also be evoked with attenuated strains, sterile oedema fluid and *in vitro*-produced antigen, but not with preparations of dead organisms. It was against this background that fresh investigations were carried out into the pathogenesis of anthrax in the early 1950s in the UK, USA, and the USSR.

In vivo **approach: experimental anthrax in the guinea pig** The fresh thrust of the work at The Microbiological Research Establishment, Porton was to examine organisms and their products derived from *in vivo* sources in suitably designed biological tests. Anthrax bacilli were injected into the thoracic and peritoneal cavities of guinea pigs. From both cavities, organisms and exudates were recovered; the latter were combined with plasma from infected animals and were regarded as a source of extracellular factors secreted by the organisms *in vivo*. Some of the different properties of the *in vivo* derived organisms are summarized in Table 6.

Table 6 Properties of *Bacillus anthracis* and its derivatives grown *in vivo* and *in vitro*

	Organisms *in vitro*	Organisms *in vivo*
Possession of capsules	$\pm$	$+++$
Susceptibility to phagocytosis	$++$	$-$
Solubility in $(NH_4)_2CO_3$	$-$	$++$

Plasma and exudates from both cavities (PE), the product obtained by dissolving organisms in ammonium carbonate (ACE), and extracts of organisms obtained with ballotini glass beads (BE) were all non-toxic when injected intraperitoneally into guinea pigs. Skin tests revealed that only PE produced any significant effect— a transient oedema. No evidence for a lethal anthrax toxin was obtained. In subsequent experiments guinea pigs were infected intradermally, and at 12 h from death the number of bacteria rose from 3×10^5 to 1×10^9 chains/ml blood. If specific antiserum or, better, streptomycin was administered at or before the time that the bacterial burden reached 0.3 per cent of the terminal level, the guinea pigs would be saved. If given after this point, the guinea pigs died even though a massive reduction in bacterial numbers was achieved. This proved the non-essentiality of the bacteraemia and suggested a toxic factor as the cause of death; the latter was duly found.

At the 'point of no return', most organisms were found in the spleen, but later the majority were found in the blood. Quantitative and qualitative analyses of blood from infected animals suggested that animals were dying of secondary oligaemic shock (see Chapter 6), as judged by the composite physiological disturbances observed. There was a loss of blood (up to 25 per cent at 1.5 h before death) and a dramatic drop in blood pressure from 8 h before death. There was evidence for fluid leakage to the site of infection and later, haemorrhage. During the final 6 h the body temperature dropped from 37 to 31°C. Carbohydrate metabolism was affected: an initial pathological rise in glucose was followed by a terminal hypoglycaemia due to bacterial metabolism. Electrolytic imbalances in plasma were observed: pH, Na^+, HCO_3^- fell; K^+, Mg^{2+} rose. There was also histopathological and biochemical evidence of renal failure. These features are characteristic of secondary shock. The Porton group showed that sterile blood from doomed guinea pigs reproduced the same syndrome in, and killed, uninfected guinea pigs; this lethal effect was specifically neutralizable with antisera. Presumably the earlier failure to find the toxin in PE was due to its dilution or inactivation by the exudates, which together with plasma, constituted PE.

Isolation of synergistic toxin complex At this time, protein separation technology was in its infancy and consequently the early attempts to isolate and purify the lethal toxin highlighted by experimental pathology were hampered by the lack of good physico-chemical separation techniques. For example, initial experiments involving heavy metal salts for differential precipitation of protein resulted in loss of toxicity. Even in the absence of such inactivating substances, ultra-centrifugation of crude plasma yielded a pellet and supernatant, both of which were non-toxic. However, mixing pellet and supernatant resulted in reconstitution of toxic activity, thus demonstrating the existence of at least 2 factors (pellet, I; supernatant, II) which comprised a synergistic toxic mixture.

Confirmation of the key findings relating to the composition of the toxin came from *in vitro* studies. When Thorne, Molnar and Strange, in 1960, produced the toxin *in vitro* and sterilized it by passage through a glass filter, only factor II was obtained. Factor I was adsorbed to the sintered glass but could be desorbed by washing it with alkaline solutions; adsorption of factor I was prevented by addition of serum before filtration. Also, Klein's group at Fort Dietrich also isolated the synergistic toxin from the blood of monkeys dying of experimental anthrax; a most important finding because this observation in primates increased the relevance of the work done on small animals as a model of the human situation.

Further fractionation studies by the Porton group revealed that purified I + II caused more oedema in guinea pig skin tests than did crude toxic plasma. Further search revealed factor III, which enhanced lethality and depressed oedema production, completing, in 1963, a picture summarized in Table 7.

Table 7 Properties of the 3-factor toxin

Factor	Oedema in skin (rabbit)	Lethality (mice)	Immunity (guinea pig)
I	−	−	−
II	−	−	+++
III	−	−	−
I+II	+++	+	++++
I + III	−	−	+
II + III	−	++	++
I + II + III	++	++++	++

By 1968, the American workers had obtained more purified preparations of all three factors and described some important differences; these were partially reflected in their choice of nomenclature. Factor II was designated protective antigen (PA), which agrees with Table 7; it is possible that the I + III combination, which was weakly protective, was contaminated with immunogenic traces of II. Factor I became oedema factor (EF) since, in combination with II, it produced oedema in guinea pigs; this combination was not lethal to rats. Factor III became lethal factor (LF) since in combination with II it was highly lethal for rats; again, the low lethality of I + II could be explained by trace contamination with III or inherent differences between rats and mice. However, some other differences were obtained which are not so easy to explain. For example, so-called PA (Factor II) protected guinea pigs against spore challenge but not rats against spores or toxin; in contrast, LF (Factor III) protected both guinea pigs and rats against spore challenge and rats against toxin. This immunogenic role of Factor III *per se* disagrees with UK findings. All three factors are proteins (probably not 'simple' proteins); factor I is probably a chelating agent, and no enzymic activity has been associated with any of the factors.

It would be fascinating to reopen this problem in the present climate of enquiry since new conceptual frameworks and fractionation techniques have been developed since work terminated in the late 60s. Using highly purified factors, many of the controversies about the pathophysiology, immunogenicity, and species variation shown by this complex toxin could be resolved.

Role of toxin in disease: pathophysiology Before summarizing this aspect it is important to remember that toxigenicity *per se* does not confer full virulence on anthrax bacilli. To synthesize a lethal dose of toxin, organisms must establish an initial bridgehead from which they can grow and spread. To succeed they need to be capsulated as well as toxigenic. The poly-D-glutamic acid present in the capsule prevents phagocytosis of organisms and the toxin actually destroys white cells. This explains why the Sterne strain, which is used as a live vaccine, is immunogenic; it is non-capsulated but is toxigenic and succeeds in producing an immunogenic dose of toxin before it is eliminated by the vaccinated host.

Several problems face the experimental pathologist in seeking to correlate the pathophysiology of intoxication and infection. First, in infected animals toxin is released in small and then in increasing amounts during bacterial multiplication and invasion, in contrast to diphtheria, tetanus or cholera, in which the causative organisms remain localized. The lethal effects are thus exerted on a progressively weakened animal, whereas in intoxication experiments, large doses are injected into healthy animals. Second, we know nothing about the dynamics and regulation of production of the three factors *in vivo* and little about the optimum combination of the factors or the order in which they must act for maximum lethal effect; it has been suggested that factor II is most rapidly removed from the circulation (fixed to target sites?) and is the means of fixing other factors at the site of action. Third, there are differences between species in their reaction to toxin. The mouse, guinea pig, rabbit, chimpanzee, rhesus monkey, dog, and rat have all been challenged with toxin but the rat (at least the Fisher strain 344) responds quite differently from the rest; it is relatively very resistant to infection and highly sensitive to toxin (factor III in particular) and exhibits atypical pathology in that toxin induces marked pulmonary oedema. Nevertheless, American workers used rats in much of their work.

Until 1968, when active research stopped, there was major disagreement between the British and American workers about the pathophysiological action of anthrax toxin. In only two species—guinea pig and monkey—were the effects of toxin and infection correlated. The British group showed that injection of toxin reproduced the major changes seen in infected animals and interpreted the primary site of action to be capillaries, whose permeability was altered, thus inducing secondary oligaemic (or hypovolaemic) shock (see Chapter 6). The American group, however, claimed that massive oedema and blood fluid loss were observed only in the rat and that secondary shock was not the cause of death in other animals. Additionally they claimed that in primates and rats, heart rate *and blood pressure* remain remarkably constant until shortly before death, which if correct would tend to argue against the secondary shock hypothesis at least in these species. The American workers believed that, at least in monkeys and rats, the primary effect of anthrax toxin is on the central nervous system with no overt histopathology in neural or other tissues. The wide range of changes observed were thought to be non-specific and the result of disfunction of the central nervous system, the primary effect being on the respiratory system.

Thus, in conclusion, different workers disagree about nomenclature, the basis of immunity in the guinea pig, and the primary cause of death within and between species. These problems may be solved by use of highly purified trace-labelled factors and the same strain of each species of experimental animal by different laboratories.

Enterotoxins

Staphylococcal enterotoxins Although relatively uncommon in the UK, staphylococcal food poisoning accounts for over 40 per cent of all cases of food poisoning in the United States. The disease is characterized by vomiting and diarrhoea commencing 1–6 h after consumption of contaminated food, especially dairy produce. Symptoms usually last no longer than 24 h and death is extremely rare.

Like botulism, staphylococcal food poisoning is commonly caused by the ingestion of food containing preformed toxins, known collectively as the staphylococcal enterotoxins. The enterotoxins have been comprehensively reviewed by Bergdoll *et al* (1974). They are a heterogeneous group of single-chain globular proteins, of molecular weight between 28 000 and 35 000 daltons, secreted by certain strains of *Staphylococcus aureus*. Six serologically distinct types (A, B, C_1, C_2, D and E) of enterotoxin have so far been recognized and, as judged by isoelectric focusing, heterogeneity exists within types A, B and C_2. No satisfactory suggestion has been forwarded to explain this heterogeneity, but, as in the case of *Clostridium perfringens* α-toxin, it is likely to reflect post-translational modifications of the molecules.

Because of the short duration and the non-fatal nature of the illness, no details are known of the effects of staphylococcal enterotoxins on particular organs and tissues in man. Much of what is known of the pathogenesis of the disease and the mode of action of the enterotoxins has been determined mainly in primates. In the monkey, oral challenge with staphylococcal enterotoxins causes vomiting, diarrhoea, and an acute inflammatory response in the gastric mucosa and small intestine. However, these effects, especially vomiting, are also observed when animals are injected intravenously with enterotoxins. Thus, these toxins cannot be considered to be classical enterotoxins, like cholera toxin or the *Escherichia coli* enterotoxins, because they do not act directly on intestinal cells. The toxin activates receptors on the abdominal viscera, the stimulus reaching the vomiting centre *via* the vagus nerve. Thus the toxins can be considered to be neurotoxins.

The molecular basis for the diarrhoeagenic effect of these toxins has yet to be elucidated. Enterotoxin B enhances fluid secretion in the small intestine of the rat and, like cholera toxin, does not affect glucose absorption, indicating that the structural integrity of the intestinal mucosa is not impaired. However, the short circuit current across the mucosa remains unchanged, suggesting that enterotoxin B does not cause fluid secretion by elevating cyclic AMP levels in the mucosal cells.

In contrast however, Huang and his colleagues using an unlikely experimental animal, the flounder, reported that staphylococcal enterotoxins induce changes in short circuit current in stripped mucosal segments and increase Na^+ and Cl^- efflux, suggesting that staphylococcal enterotoxins, like cholera toxin, have an effect on adenylate cyclase, though this has yet to be confirmed.

Apart from their gastrointestinal effects, the staphylococcal enterotoxins have been reported to suppress murine spleen cell antibody response and to induce polyclonal stimulation of human and murine lymphocytes. The relevance of such immunological effects to pathogenicity is uncertain and will not be discussed further here. However, such effects are not directly related to enterotoxic activity because heat destroys enterotoxicity but not mitogenic effects of the proteins.

Clostridium perfringens enterotoxin Unlike food poisoning due to *Clostridium botulinum* and *Staphylococcus aureus*, which is caused by the ingestion of food contaminated with preformed toxin, gastroenteritis or the more severe and quite distinct disease enteritis necroticans ('pig bel') caused by *C. perfringens* is the result of enteric infection and release of toxins in the gut. It is important to distinguish the two types of disease and the toxins responsible for them.

C. perfringens was first suspected of causing food poisoning is the 1890s, when Klein in Germany and Andrewes in London isolated the organism from food thought to have caused illness. In 1949, Zeissler and Rassfeld-Sternberg investigated an outbreak of a rare, severe and often fatal haemorrhagic enteric disease called 'enteritis necroticans' (discussed later in this chapter). They isolated from suspect food and patients' faeces a strain of *C. perfringens* which they designated type F, but which is now considered to be a heat-stable variant of type C.

In 1953, using human volunteers, Hobbs identified *C. perfringens* type A as the cause of the much more common but less severe form of food poisoning. Cravitz and Gillmore had previously shown that ingestion of sterile culture filtrates of *C. perfringens* isolated from cases of food poisoning caused nausea, stomach cramps, and vomiting in humans, suggesting the involvement of a toxin. Further investigation of the determinants of *C. perfringens* food poisoning was hampered by the fact that experimental illness could not at first be produced in laboratory animals. Then, in the late 1960s, using cultures of the organism, Hauschild and Duncan produced experimental diarrhoea in lambs and rabbits respectively.

Duncan then showed that sporulating cultures of *C. perfringens* could cause fluid secretion in ligated segments of rabbit ileum. Hauschild and colleagues later showed that the toxin was identical to a previously reported guinea pig erythemal factor and proposed that the erythrogenic response (following intradermal injection) be employed as a convenient assay for enterotoxicity in isolates of *C. perfringens*.

The enterotoxin has been purified, is a protein of molecular weight 35 000 daltons, and a structural component of the spore. Recently, an apparently identical enterotoxin has been isolated from strains of *C. perfringens* type C, implicated in the much more severe disease, enteritis necroticans.

The mechanism of action of the enterotoxin is at present unknown. Like cholera and *E. coli* enterotoxins, it causes diarrhoea by reversing the net flow of Na^+, Cl^-, and water from absorption to secretion. However, unlike these toxins, it does not affect intracellular cyclic AMP levels in the gut or in cells in culture. It has been reported that glucose absorption in the gut is inhibited by the toxin, indicating that the net fluid and ion losses are due to decreased absorption rather than increased secretion. This view is strengthened by the recent observation that *C. perfringens* type A enterotoxin inhibits active transport of amino acids across the membrane of isolated rat hepatocytes. This inhibition of active transport is dose-dependent and abolished by specific antitoxin. Kinetics of inhibition indicate that the site of toxin action is not intracellular but at the membrane.

Toxins of known importance but action not known

***Bacillus cereus* enterotoxins** Although *Bacillus cereus* has been implicated in food poisoning since the turn of the century, it was not until 1955, when the Norwegian, Hauge, deliberately consumed a portion of vanilla sauce containing 92×10^6 organisms per ml, that it was conclusively shown to cause food-borne disease. The 'classical' form of *B. cereus* gastroenteritis, as experienced by Hauge, is characterized by diarrhoea, abdominal pain and cramps some 8–16 h after the ingestion of food contaminated with the organism. However, only rarely is illness accompanied by vomiting.

Culture filtrates of isolates from cases of gastroenteritis were shown by Goepfert and his colleagues in the early 1970s to contain a protein enterotoxin, of molecular weight approximately 50 000 daltons which, like cholera toxin, causes fluid secretion in ligated rabbit ileal loops by activating adenylate cyclase. This toxin, which also increased vascular permeability in the skin of rabbits and is lethal to mice when injected parenterally, may be responsible for the complete disease syndrome.

Since the early 1970s, however, there have been numerous reports of outbreaks of 'atypical' *B. cereus* food poisoning, often associated with rice dishes obtained from Chinese 'take away' restaurants. This illness differs from the classical gastroenteritis in that consumption of contaminated food is followed 1–5 h later by acute nausea and vomiting, but not diarrhoea. Thus the term '*B. cereus* food poisoning' obviously encompasses two quite distinct clinical syndromes, which pointed to the existence of at least two enterotoxins. This belief was strengthened, in 1976, by the observation that oral administration to rhesus monkeys of *B. cereus* isolated from gastroenteritis caused fluid secretion in ligated ileal loops and diarrhoea, but no vomiting. In contrast, *B. cereus* isolated from fried rice caused a negative ileal loop reaction and vomiting, but no diarrhoea. Moreover, the organism caused vomiting only when grown on rice. These experiments suggested that, while organisms causing gastroenteritis possess a diarrhoeagenic toxin, the vomiting disease may be caused by a separate emetic toxin. Such a toxin has since been recognized and has a molecular weight ≤ 5000 daltons, is heat-stable, and is probably spore-associated.

Further work by Turnbull led to the discovery of isolates of *B. cereus* which caused yet another pathological syndrome. Culture filtrates of these organisms which were isolated from cases of diarrhoea, vomiting and wound infections, induce disruption and necrosis of the intestinal mucosa when injected into ligated rabbit ileal loops. However, whether this is caused by a single toxin or several toxic substances acting in concert has yet to be established.

Thus the spectrum of food-borne disease caused by *B. cereus* is broad, as is the range of potentially toxic substances known to be elaborated by this organism (Table 8), and while a definite role in pathogenesis may be ascribed for the diarrhoeagenic and emetic toxins, the position of the other toxic factors is less clearly defined. For example, the extensive necrotic intestinal lesions produced by some strains of *B. cereus* could conceivably be caused by the diarrhoeagenic toxin or any of the remaining toxins, either individually or in combination.

***Shigella* enterotoxins** Shigellosis is characterized by acute diarrhoea accompanied by febrile colitis involving necrosis of intestinal epithelium (dysentery). The disease is classically caused by *Shigella dysenteriae* type 1, but may also be caused by other shigellae, such as *S. boydii*, *S. sonnei* and *S. flexneri*.

In 1903, Conradi demonstrated that sterile culture filtrates of *S. dysenteriae* 1 contained a neurotoxic component which, when injected into susceptible animals, caused limb paralysis and death. Further investigation showed that injection of the

Table 8 Extracellular toxins and other factors of *Bacillus cereus*

| Product | Physico-chemical properties | | | Additional biological properties |
	Molecular weight	Number of electrophoretic forms	pI	
diarrhoeagenic toxin (vascular permeability factor, mouse lethal factor)	55–60 000	1	4.85	causes diarrhoea by activation of adenylate cyclase. alters vascular permeability when injected intradermally in rabbits. lethal to mice. may be necrotic.
emetic toxin	≤ 5 000	—	—	vomiting on oral administration probably not protein sporulation-specific?
thiol-activated haemolysin (cereolysin)	50–60 000	2 (oxidised and reduced)	6.3–6.7	membrane-damaging may be lethal to mice when injected intravenously in large quantities.
2nd haemolysin	—	—	5.0	little knowledge of this at present
phospholipases C: phosphatidyl choline specific	23 000	1	8.1	non haemolytic
phosphatidyl inositol specific	29 000	1	—	
2nd mouse lethal factor	—	1	6.6	cereolysin?
toxin of Ezepchuk and Fluer	55–60 000	1	—	vomiting in cats. lethal to mice and rabbits relationship to other toxins unknown

Data compiled from Turnbull P. C. B. *et al* (1979) *Am. J. Clin. Nut.* 32: 219.

neurotoxin preparation into rabbits produced lesions in the mucosa of the caecum superficially identical with those caused by live organisms in human shigellosis. However, subsequent work by Olitsky and Kliger, in 1920, indicated that the neurotoxic preparations in fact contained two biologically active constituents: a protein toxin responsible for the neurological lesions and a lipopolysaccharide endotoxin believed to be responsible for the lesions in the gut. Because the neurotoxin did not cause lesions similar to those observed in human shigellosis, a role for this toxin in the pathogenicity of *S. dysenteriae* 1 was discounted.

The discoveries by Keusch and his colleagues in the early 1970s resurrected the question of the role of toxins in shigella infections. They partially purified from culture filtrates of *S. dysenteriae* 1 a protein toxin which in ligated segments of rabbit ileum caused fluid accumulation and histopathological changes in the intestinal mucosa which resembled the early lesions observed after oral challenge with live bacteria. This toxic preparation, when injected into mice, also caused neurological lesions of the type described by Conradi. (An apparently identical toxin has since been isolated from *S. flexneri* type 2A.)

Further work showed the *S. dysenteriae* 1 toxin to cause cytotoxic changes in HeLa cells *in vitro*, probably by inhibition of protein synthesis, and Keusch used this as a very sensitive and convenient assay during purification procedures. In 1975 toxic preparations were discovered which could be resolved by isoelectric focusing into two components: one (pI = 6.0) possessing cytotoxic activity and the other (pI = 7.2) exhibiting cytotoxicity, neurotoxicity, and enterotoxicity. It has been suggested that the cytotoxic protein (pI = 6.0) is a sub-unit or sub-component of the larger protein (pI = 7.2) though this has yet to be confirmed. Very recently, Keusch and Jacewicz presented persuasive evidence that shigella toxin reaches its target site in HeLa cells *via* endocytosis during which it probably undergoes processing and activation.

Incubation of partially purified shigella toxin with HeLa or mammalian liver cell membranes reduces the toxicity of the preparation for HeLa cells, indicating that these membrane fragments possess specific receptors for the toxin, which is adsorbed out of the toxic preparation. Binding inhibition studies suggest that the toxin receptor contains on oligomeric $\beta1 \rightarrow 4$ linked N-acetyl-D-glucosamine determinant. Armed with this knowledge, Keusch purified small quantities of toxin by affinity chromatography using chitin oligosaccharide linked to a suitable matrix. The protein thus purified has a molecular weight of approximately 70 000 daltons and possesses cytotoxic and neurotoxic activities. The enterotoxic activity of the protein was not determined, possibly because of the relative insensitivity of the assay.

The mechanism of the diarrhoeagenic response is still unknown. An obvious suggestion has been that, like cholera toxin, shigella toxin exerts its enterotoxic effects by stimulation of adenylate cyclase. Formal's group has showed that activation of adenylate cyclase in rabbit ileal mucosa by shigella toxin injected into ligated ileal loops can be observed only if ATP concentrations far greater than those required to demonstrate activation by cholera toxin are employed. This diminishes the possibility that shigella toxin induces intestinal secretion primarily by activation of adenylate cyclase and suggests that net fluid and electrolyte efflux may be mediated by as yet undefined mechanisms.

The relationship of the adenylate cyclase activating toxin to the enterotoxic component isolated by Keusch is unknown, but limited evidence suggests that they may be different. A 'toxin' has recently been isolated which causes morphological changes in chinese hamster ovary (CHO) cells *in vitro*—a change mediated by activation of adenylate cyclase and also brought about by cholera toxin—but which lacks neurotoxicity and is not lethal to mice. In contrast, the enterotoxin isolated by Keusch possesses cytotoxic and neurotoxic activities. The role of these toxic activities in disease is still in doubt, however. Many workers see the ability of *S. dysenteriae* 1 to invade the epithelial cells of the colon as the prime virulence factor of the organism. Two independent studies have shown that while invasive non-toxigenic variants of *S. dysenteriae* cause clinical shigellosis in human volunteers, non-invasive toxigenic strains are harmless. Keusch has argued, however, that failure to demonstrate toxin *in vitro* does not mean that toxin is not produced *in vivo* and, moreover, has shown that one allegedly non-toxigenic strain used in these studies not only produces cytotoxin under appropriate conditions *in vitro* but also *in vivo* as judged by antibody response to cytotoxin in infected humans.

So, the role of toxins in shigellosis is still unclear. However, the fact that shigellosis involves both diarrhoea and necrosis of mucosal tissue, and that *S. dysenteriae* 1 elaborates a toxin or toxins capable of producing both these symptoms, is persuasive evidence in support of these toxins as important virulence factors.

Exfoliatin and the staphylococcal scalded skin syndrome The disease now known as staphylococcal scalded skin syndrome (SSSS) was first reported in 1878 by Ritter von Rittershain, who described nearly three hundred cases of what he termed '*dermatitis exfoliativa neonatorum*' in newly born babies at his foundling hospital in Prague.

The disease is characterized by a region of erythema which usually begins around the mouth and, in 1–2 days, extends over the whole body. During this period, small yellowish exudative lesions often appear. The most striking feature of the disease, however, is that the epidermis, although apparently healthy, can be displaced and wrinkled like the skin of a ripe peach by the slightest pressure. Soon large areas of the epidermis become lifted by a layer of serous fluid and peel at the slightest touch. Large areas of the body rapidly become denuded in this way and the symptoms resemble those of massive scalding. As the denuded areas dry, however, the epithelium is replaced. In 1898, Winternitz isolated *Staphylococcus aureus* and *S. albus* from patients suffering from what had come to be known as Ritter's disease; in 1970 it was finally confirmed to be a rare manifestation of staphylococcal infection.

Since the mid 1950s there have been several reports of a seemingly identical disease in adults. However, in many cases this disease (named toxic epidermal necrolysis; TEN) is due not to staphylococci, but to a hypersensitive reaction to several drugs. There are, moreover, distinct histological differences between SSSS and allergic TEN, and to avoid further confusion the term SSSS has been adopted for the bacterial disease.

Winternitz remarked, in 1898, upon the frequency with which *S. aureus* and *S. albus* could be isolated from patients with SSSS, an observation which underwent considerable consolidation in the years up to 1955, when Parker presented evidence which strongly implicated *S. aureus* of phage group II as the causative organism. However, the lack of a suitable animal model meant that an unequivocal causal relationship could not be established. Then, in 1970, Melish and Glasgow showed that subcutaneous injection into newborn mice of group II staphylococci isolated from cases of SSSS caused a very similar disease in these animals. Thus, the missing animal model had been found and the relationship between staphylococci and SSSS was established.

This important breakthrough enabled Arbuthnott and Kapral independently to confirm, in 1971, that SSSS is caused by the action of a specific toxin elaborated by staphylococci. Using the newborn mouse model, they showed that partially purified, sterile, soluble products of group II staphylococci could bring about experimental SSSS, and it was later shown that these effects could be blocked by specific antitoxin.

The toxin responsible for SSSS, often called exfoliatin, was long thought to be produced almost exclusively by phage group II staphylococci and, as for some other bacterial toxins, the gene for toxin synthesis to be located on a plasmid, but this need not always be so. Exfoliatin from phage group II staphylococci was purified in several laboratories in the early 1970s and shown to be a protein of molecular weight approximately 25–30 000 daltons which is inactivated by incubation below pH 4.0, but survives heating to 60°C for one hour. Isoelectric focusing of partially purified toxin gave a major band of activity at pH 7.1, but a minor band of activity at pH 6.2 was observed. Treatment of the toxin with urea failed to remove the minor band of toxic activity, indicating that there are two distinct but serologically identical forms of the toxin. Then, in 1974, Kondo and his associates isolated exfoliatin from non-phage group II staphylococci. This protein was less heat-stable and immunologically distinct from that of group II organisms but had a similar molecular weight and could be purified using the same experimental conditions. Recently, Arbuthnott's group, using more sensitive separation and assay procedures showed that although all epidermolysis-producing staphylococci synthesize a chromosomally coded toxin designated serotype i, they may also elaborate a plasmid-coded, heat-labile, immunologically distinct toxin molecule designated serotype ii (the toxin recognized by Kondo). Moreover, synthesis of exfoliatin serotypes i and ii is by no means confined to phage group II staphylococci.

The principal pathological feature of the disease is cell separation at the epidermis, more specifically, *within* the epidermis, followed by massive denuding of the body surface. The intra-epidermal splitting, a feature which distinguishes SSSS from allergic TEN, occurs at the *stratum granulosum* (the layer of cells destined to become the dead, flattened cells of the skin surface Fig. 14;) and involves minimal necrosis. The mechanism by which exfoliatin achieves intra-epidermal splitting is not known, but all available evidence suggests that it is an extracellular, non-cytotoxic process. One suggestion is that the intercellular bubbles might contain an enzyme or pro-enzyme which is released or activated by exfoliatin, and which then acts on the nearest desmosome to cause splitting. This hypothesis also accounts for the unique specificity of the toxin for cells of the *stratum granulosum*, since only the spaces between these cells have been shown to possess such bubbles.

Clostridial toxins

In this section we will look at clostridial toxins, other than those considered previously, which are at least associated with, if not important determinants of, several diseases of both man and animals. The clostridial genus comprises a large number of toxigenic species, some of which are known to produce several toxins,

Bacterial Toxins

extracellular enzymes, and other factors which are as yet recognized only by a letter of the Greek alphabet or as unidentified lines in immunoanalytical gels. In Table 2 we presented a summary of this situation with an indication of some of the properties of the better known toxins and enzymes, and of the manner in which such information is exploited taxonomically.

We have subdivided this section according to causative organisms and the diseases they produce in man and in animals, and given a brief description of the essential features of the disease to facilitate discussion of possible toxic factors important in the genesis of lesions or death. No attempt will be made to describe

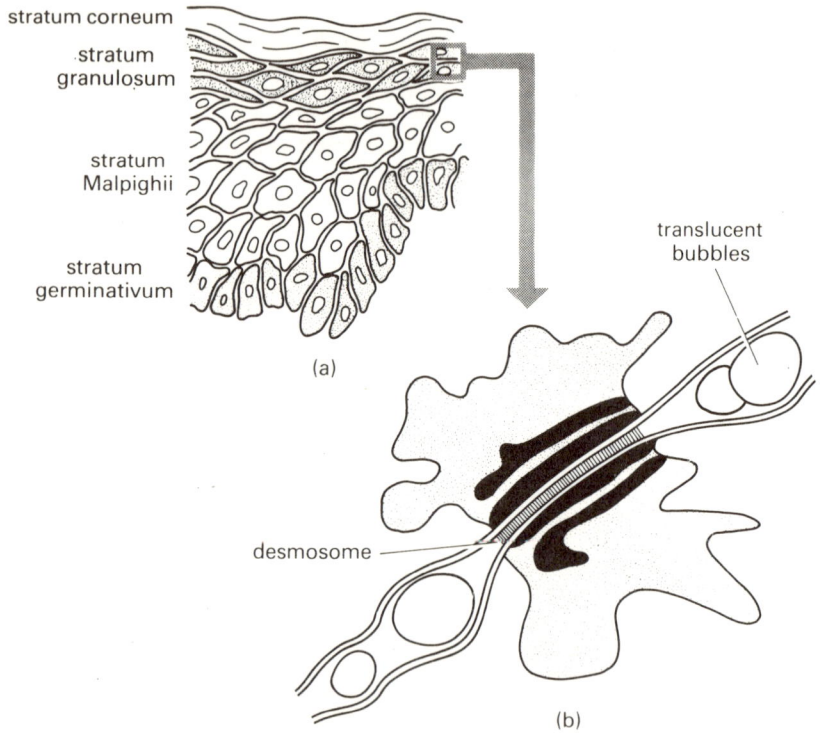

(a)

(b)

Figure 14 The site of action of exfoliatin, showing the location of the stratum granulosum in the epidermis (a) and the structures to be found at the cell junctions (b). Electron microscopy reveals that the individual cells of the *stratum granulosum* are attached to each other by specialized cell membrane thickenings called desmosomes, and that the spaces between the cells are filled with material containing small translucent 'bubbles'. Treatment of tissue with exfoliatin causes these bubbles to disappear rapidly, followed by a widening of the intercellular gap and splitting of desmosomes, with each half of the organelle remaining with its parent cells. Thus a large cleft is soon formed between the layers of cells.

(Reprinted with permission from Lillibridge, C. B., *Pediatrics* (1972), **50**, 728–738.)

every disease in man or animals associated with clostridia; only those will be selected which best serve to illustrate the involvement of some recognizable toxins. In the case of sheep diseases—lamb dysentery, struck, enterotoxaemia, black disease, braxy, black quarter—some of the best evidence for implicating relevant toxins comes from field studies using multivalent vaccines against all those diseases and, therefore, this aspect will be discussed at the end of this section under 'Immunity to clostridial diseases'. The descriptive pathology of the clostridial infections of animals has been taken largely from the excellent article by Roberts (1959).

Clostridium perfringens type C; pig bel in man This disease is rare in developed societies but until recently it was a major public health hazard in Papua, New Guinea. There are four factors responsible for the disease: the ubiquity of *C. perfringens* type C in the soil and faeces of man and pigs; the relatively low immunogenicity of β-toxoids in young children, the group most at risk; the high carbohydrate, low protein nature of the staple diet; and the sporadic consumption of large quantities of pork on occasions of celebration. The latter dietary change promotes a proliferation of clostridia in the intestine which may lead to intestinal gangrene and death.

Recent work, involving workers from New Guinea, Australia, and the UK, suggests that β-toxin is the most important toxin elaborated by *C. perfringens* type C and that this damages the mucosa, reduces mobility of the villi and causes more bacteria to become attached to the villi. More toxin is absorbed and the mucosa and underlying intestinal wall become necrotic, leading to death in many cases. The influence of diet is additionally important in that low protein diets causes decreased secretion of pancreatic proteolytic enzymes and sweet potato contains a trypsin inhibitor. These conditions promote the survival of β-toxin which is highly sensitive to proteolytic inactivation.

Immunization with β-toxoid preparations has dramatically lowered the incidence of this fatal disease in children without any major cultural changes in the population. With changes in the latter the disease would predictably disappear.

Clostridium novyi types A and B; gas gangrene in man As was pointed out in Chapter 3, gas gangrene in man may be caused by several bacterial species separately or in concert. These include *Clostridium perfringens* type A, *C. novyi* types A and B, and *C. septicum*; *C. perfringens* and its α-toxin have already been discussed at some length. Far less is known about *C. novyi* and *C. septicum* and their toxins in the context of gas gangrene in man. In contrast, much is known about the role these organisms play in diseases of animals and it was against this background of knowledge and successes achieved in preventing these diseases by use of formalin-prepared toxoids, that Boyd and co-workers devised experiments (already described in the context of *C. perfringens* α-toxin; Chapter 3, page 43) to test the prophylactic value of appropriate antitoxins in preventing clinical gas gangrene induced by high velocity bullet wounds in sheep. We must emphasize that this was a model for human gas gangrene as experienced under wartime conditions; sheep do get gas gangrene (black quarter) but not by this method(!) and rarely with *C. novyi*, but nearly always with *C. chauvoei*. Using this model, it was shown that gas gangrene caused by *C. novyi* could be prevented by active immunization with *C. novyi* α-toxoid preparations or passive administration of α-antitoxin if the latter were given soon after infection.

Clostridium difficile; **pseudomembranous colitis in man** This disease has recently been recognized as toxin-mediated and is currently being actively investigated. It occurs in patients who have been treated with certain antibiotics before or after major gut surgery. This creates conditions favourable for the growth of *C. difficile*, which is not normally active in the gut of healthy persons (it may be absent), and the elaboration of a toxin which is believed to be responsible for the diarrhoea and death in severely incapacitated patients. It is neutralized by antitoxin raised to *C. sordelli* toxin and is toxic to cultured cells, but little is known about its nature or mode of action.

Clostridium perfringens **type B; lamb dysentery** This is an acute, fatal disease of young lambs occurring during the first week of life (often during the second or third day) and caused by absorption of toxin(s) generated by *C. perfringens* type B in the small intestine. The principal pathological feature is damage to the wall of the intestine, which may vary from hyperaemia to deep ulceration, and the presence of *C. perfringens* type B and/or β- and ε-toxins. However, in the most acute cases there may be no apparent abnormality. The factors which predispose lambs to infection are not known and the disease is not readily reproducible by oral feeding of culture filtrates.

Clostridium perfringens **type C; struck in sheep** This disease (also described as strike, haemorrhagic enterotoxaemia or enterotoxaemia (type C)) is common in unprotected adult sheep in the Romney marshes of Kent but rare in other areas in the world. The pathological changes observed differ markedly from other enterotoxaemias and include enteritis, sometimes abomasitis, ulceration in the small intestine in some cases, contraction of the walls of the small intestine, extensive transudations in the peritoneal cavity, marked prominence and haemorrhage of the peritoneal blood vessels and, less frequently, transudations in the thoracic cavity and pericardium. Toxin is generally present in the abomasum or in the intestinal contents.

Clostridium perfringens **type D; enterotoxaemia in sheep** This is another acute fatal disease, sometimes called pulpy kidney disease or overeating disease. The most constant lesion is sub-endocardial haemorrhage around the mitral valve. There is also excess fluid in the pericardial sac. At death the kidney may show small degenerative changes which become progressively worse until the organ becomes soft and, on removal of the capsule, the parenchyma is readily washed away; this is almost certainly a *post mortem* change. *C. perfringens* type D ε-toxin or its protoxin are recoverable from intestinal contents.

Bullen (1970) provides an excellent description of experimentally induced disease. Under normal or nutritionally low-plane dietary conditions, introduction of large numbers of *C. perfringens* type D over a long period into the duodenum of a sheep does not cause overt disease. However, when a rich diet is suddenly fed *ad lib*, sheep overeat to the extent that the microbial flora of the rumen cannot adapt sufficiently quickly, resulting in an overspill of unfermented starch into the small intestine. Under such conditions, huge numbers of *C. perfringens* type D are generated *and maintained* and produce lethal levels of ε-toxin, which is absorbed due to an alteration in intestinal permeability. The disease is also reproducible by administration of sterile toxic filtrates.

The altered permeability is demonstrable in mice and sheep by detecting increased levels of marker proteins (unrelated antitoxins) in the blood after oral or intra-duodenal administration of sterile culture filtrates to mice or sheep respectively. Two factors are responsible for this change, at least in mice: ε-toxin, whose effects are neutralizable by specific antitoxin, and another heat-stable factor which appears to increase the ε-toxin-induced permeability. The introduction into the duodenum of organisms immediately after change to a rich diet or of high doses of sterile culture filtrate kills sheep with the principal signs of the natural disease, in which animals die within $1\frac{1}{4}$ h of the development of typical nervous convulsions. These experimental studies on *C. perfringens* type D enterotoxaemia fit well with field studies, which strongly suggest that this disease is often associated with a rapid movement of unprotected sheep from poor to rich pasture.

Clostridium novyi **type B; black disease of sheep** Black disease (infectious necrotic hepatitis), is an acute infectious disease of sheep (occasionally cattle) caused by the absorption of toxin elaborated by the organism in necrotic foci in the liver, and is nearly always associated with invasion of the liver by immature liver flukes. How *C. novyi* gets to the liver in the first place is not known but it is readily demonstrable in livers of normal sheep in areas where the disease is prevalent. Experimental reproduction in guinea pigs of a similar disease is possible by the combined action of *C. novyi* spores and liver fluke infestation. It is without doubt a toxaemia (almost certainly α-toxaemia), since organisms can only be isolated from necrotic foci in the liver.

The main features of this disease in sheep can be reproduced easily in mice and guinea pigs with cultures or culture filtrates. In addition to complex changes occurring in the liver, subcutaneous blood vessels are engorged and this, together with extensive subcutaneous oedema which becomes heavily blood-stained as the carcass ages, accounts for the popular name of the disease. The peritoneal cavity and the pericardial sac contain exudates and there is subcutaneous and intermuscular exudate extending along the floor of the abdomen.

Clostridium novyi **type D; redwater disease in cattle** This rapidly fatal disease in cattle is similar to, and regarded by some as an atypical manifestation of, black disease. The characteristic lesions include jaundice, subcutaneous haemorrhage and oedema, excess thoracic and pericardial fluid, intense haemorrhagic enteritis, and haemorrhagic lymphadenitis. The liver is enlarged and jaundiced and invariably characterized by large anaemic infarcts caused by blockage of a branch of the portal vein; active liver fluke infestation may or may not be present. In culture this organism produces only β-toxin (Table 2) and no α-toxin. This explains the most characteristic feature of the disease, haemoglobinuria, but poses a problem. If, β-toxin is the principal lethal agent why is there no evidence for its role in type B infections? The lethal effect of type B filtrates is almost entirely due to α-toxin, despite the presence of β-toxin, and infections are prevented by active immunization with toxoids which elicit high levels of α-antitoxin. Either β-toxin, which is a phospholipase C, is not the lethal agent in redwater disease, or massive production in the liver leads to generalized permeability changes which gives rise to the characteristic oedema, haemorrhage, vascular haemolysis and death.

Injection of this organism into animals produces a gas gangrene-type disease with extensive oedematous infiltration of the subcutaneous and intramuscular connective tissue. This suggests that a factor resembling the α-toxin of types A and B may be produced *in vivo* by strains which, when typed on the basis of toxin production *in vitro*, do not produce α-toxin. These questions have never been properly resolved, nor has the highly typical liver lesion been experimentally produced. Active immunity can readily be engendered by vaccines comprising whole culture preparations, but this has not been carefully dissected serologically and, therefore, will not be discussed further.

Clostridium septicum; **braxy in sheep** The role of *C. septicum* in this acute, fatal disease is assumed because of its association with the characteristic haemorrhagic inflammatory lesion in the abomasum. The disease has not been reproduced experimentally with *C. septicum* but can be prevented by immunization with sterile toxoids derived from this organism.

Clostridium chauvoei; **black quarter in sheep and cattle** This is a gas gangrene-type infection of muscles and associated connective tissues in cattle and sheep; *C. chauvoei* is also the causative agent of parturient gas gangrene in sheep. The initiatory stimulus which activates the infection in cattle is not known, since the disease is hardly ever associated with any overt wounding. Washed spores alone do not cause disease when injected, but do in conjunction with a tissue-necrotizing agent. Thus, in the case of cattle, dormant clostridial spores may always be present in muscle and only cause disease when activated by some agency. In sheep, wounding caused by parturition, castration, tailing, shearing, vaccination, as well as accidental damage will create a focus within which *C. chauvoei* can multiply.

Guinea pigs, which are less susceptible than sheep to the effect of whole culture or toxin challenge, are used to assay vaccine or serum potency by direct challenge with live organisms when it is uneconomical to use sheep. Such tests are necessary because of the comparatively low lethality of chauvoei toxin(s): for example α-toxin is produced as part of an immunizing antigen complex but is not itself immunogenic, which makes toxin neutralization tests very difficult to carry out. Practical vaccines are based on whole cultures so will contain toxoided extracellular and also cellular material. In fact, recent failures in this field have highlighted the need for strain specificity with respect to the *C. chauvoei* component of the complex vaccine discussed in the next section.

Immunity to clostridial diseases in animals It is practical field studies on which much of our confidence is based with respect to the role in infection of the principal lethal factors known to be produced by the various clostridia discussed here. Most people are understandably aware of the dramatic success scored in the field of human prophylactic medicine. In contrast, few will be aware of the less publicized but equally remarkable successes with clostridial vaccines in the veterinary field which are responsible for the saving of many millions of pounds worth of ever-increasingly valuable livestock. The systematic study of the clostridia over many years resulted in the recognition of lethal toxins in culture filtrates which are the main basis on which highly successful prophylactic vaccines are made. Multivalent vaccines have been developed comprising products derived from cultures of *C. perfringens* types B, C and D; *C. novyi, C. septicum, C. chauvoei,* and *C. tetani.* When combined with certain adjuvants and injected by an appropriate route, they confer a very high degree of immunity (particularly to sheep) against several clinically identifiable but separate diseases.

With the exception of its *C. chauroei* and *C. tetani* components, this complex vaccine is standardized with respect to doses of the following: *C. perfringens* (types B, C, D) β and ε toxoids, *C. novyi* α-toxoid, and *C. septicum* α-toxoid. The efficacy of the vaccine is determined by the antitoxin responses elicited to these antigens and the high success rate in the field—the supreme test of any vaccine. From such observations it is inconceivable not to ascribe an important role to *C. perfringens* β- and ε-toxins, *C. novyi* α-toxin, *C. septicum* α-toxin in the pathogenesis of the diseases described; however, one cannot absolutely rule out the possibility that other factors might also play a vital or ancilliary role. These questions, as indeed questions on the site and modes of action of these toxins, will be settled only by experiments of a kind already described in this book. To do this will require an ingenuity beyond that required to conceive and execute the requisite experiments, but also one which will command resources to tackle the purely academic aspects of problems already solved practically!

In conclusion, this study of clostridial toxins highlights some fascinating problems in infectious disease. Our concern has been with terminal events, usually the lethal effects, of toxins. But of equal fascination and importance are the challenging questions of aetiology of these diseases. How and when does *C. chauvoei* get to cattle muscle in the absence of injury, or *C. novyi* to sheep liver? What are the specific inductive events which trigger, or enhance to lethal levels, toxin production in the alimentary tract to give rise to enterotoxaemia in sheep or food poisoning in man when we know that these organisms may be found in healthy individuals? Why is black disease in Australian sheep associated with *C. novyi* type B but 'big head' in Australian rams (infection of head wounds caused by butting, and not discussed in this chapter) with *C. novyi* type A, when there seems so little difference between types A and B as now classified? Why is it that *C. chauvoei* is by far the most common proven cause of black quarter (gas gangrene) in sheep and cattle, and not *C. perfringens* and *C. septicum*, even though they may be present on the same pasture land and can vigorously outgrow *C. chauvoei* in culture?

Streptococcal erythrogenic toxins

Streptococcal erythrogenic toxins are involved in the production of the characteristic rash seen in scarlet fever and hence the name and their inclusion here; however, the significance of this phenomenon in streptococcal infections is very doubtful.

Erythrogenic toxin is a low molecular weight protein produced in a complex form with hyaluronic acid, which acts as a carrier. The protein consists of two parts. One is heat-labile, carries the determinants of immunological specificity which give rise to three serotypes, A, B and C, and is responsible for primary toxicity manifestations, including pyrogenicity, low lethality, cytotoxic effects on cultured spleen macrophages, and suppression of the reticuloendothelial and immune systems. The second part is heat-stable, antigenically common to types A, B and C, and is responsible for secondary toxicity; that is, hypersensitivity effects, including skin hyperreactivity (the basis of the rash), myocardial necrosis, enhancement of pyrogenicity and lethality, and enhanced host response to other injurious agents. Thus, it is not possible to define the biological activity of 'erythrogenic' toxins without considering the immunological state of the host. An individual may suffer no reddening of the skin upon intradermal injection of erythrogenic toxin (negative Dick test) because a high neutralizing titre of antibody blocks the primary toxiphore or because of a lack of hypersensitivity to the common antigen.

Perhaps the most fascinating feature of these toxins is the manner in which they increase the sensitivity of a host to other streptococcal factors (for example, streptolysin-O) and also to Gram-negative endotoxin. The susceptibility of rabbits to endotoxin is increased 100 000 times, and adult cynomolgus monkeys die within 24 h, when injection of low levels of streptococcal toxin is followed 3 h later by an otherwise sub-lethal dose of endotoxin. Other experiments have been done in rabbits sensitized to bovine immunoglobulin. Some were injected with crude extract of a streptococcal lesion known to contain A toxin. All animals were then given an intravenous injection of the sensitizing antigen, immunoglobulin. The animals treated with streptococcal toxin either died or showed acute anaphylactic reactions, in contrast to the lack of distress in the control group.

Such observations have led to suggestions that the enhancement of susceptibility to streptolysin-O and endotoxins may not be specific, but evidence of the ability of streptococcal toxin to create a state of hypersusceptibility to a wide variety of stressful agents. Currently, there is considerable interest in mixed infections where one organism increases the severity of infection by another. Synergistic toxins (anthrax, staphylococcal leucocidin, staphylococcal γ-toxin, guinea pig plague toxin) and synergy between toxins produced by one species (staphylococcal α and δ toxins) were discussed previously: this is an example of synergy between toxins of different species (streptococcal erythrogenic toxin and endotoxin). Perhaps, in view of the high incidence of exposure of man and his domestic animals to streptococci and the facts briefly stated here, we should actively investigate possible toxin-mediated synergy in mixed infections involving streptococci.

Summary

The discovery of the synergistic toxin complex elaborated by *Bacillus anthracis* is a classic example of the analysis of the determinants of bacterial toxins *in vivo*.

Staphylococcal enterotoxins cause diarrhoea and vomiting, the latter by stimulation of the vagus nerve. *C. perfringens* enterotoxin is a protein spore component which is diarrhoegenic by virtue of inhibiting fluid uptake.

Bacillus cereus produces several toxic products, two of which, a diarrhoegenic and an emetic toxin, are involved in food poisoning. The former may act like cholera toxin.

Shigella species cause dysentery by a toxin which apparently possesses both cytotoxicity and enterotoxicity; the latter activity may be cholera-like.

Exfoliatin, responsible for the main feature of SSSS lesions, enterotoxins and α-toxin in gangrenous mastitis, are the only staphylococcal toxins known to be definitely involved in the genesis of staphylococcal diseases.

A variety of clostridial toxins are of importance in both human and veterinary diseases. Their implication as determinants of pathogenicity rests on the ability to reproduce the principal features of the respective diseases by injection of sterile culture filtrates and/or the prevention of infection by appropriate antitoxins.

References

BERGDOLL, M. S., HUANG, I. Y. & SCHANTZ, E. J. (1974). 'The chemistry of the staphylococcal enterotoxins.' *J. Agric. Food Chem.* 22: 9.

BULLEN, J. J. (1970). 'Role of toxins in host-parasite relationships.' In: *Microbial Toxins* Vol. I. p. 233. Edited by S. J. Ajl, S. Kadis and T. C. Montie. Academic Press.

DIMOND, R. L., WOLFF, H. H. & BRAUN-FALCO, O. (1977). 'The staphylococcal scalded skin syndrome.' *Brit. J. Dermatology* 96: 483.

HOBBS, B. C. (1974). '*Clostridium welchii* and *Bacillus cereus* infection and intoxication.' *Postgrad. Med. J.* 50: 597.

KEUSCH, G. T. & JACEWICZ, M. (1977). 'Pathogenesis of *Shigella* diarrhoea.' *J. Exp. Med. 146*: 535.

LINCOLN, R. E. & FISH, D. C. (1970). 'Anthrax toxin.' In: *Bacterial Toxins* Vol. III p. 361. Edited by T. C. Montie, S. Kadis, and S. J. Ajl. Academic Press.

LUCKEY, T. D. Ed. (1979). 'Intestinal microecology: Vth International Symposium.' *Am. J. Clin. Nut. 32*: No 1 pp. 105–265.

Report on conference on anthrax. (1967). *Federation proceedings 26*: No 5.

ROBERTS, R. S. (1959). In: *Infectious diseases of animals*. Vol. I. p. 160. Edited by A. W. Stableforth and I. A. Galloway. Butterworth.

SMITH, L. D. S. (1975). *The pathogenic anaerobic bacteria*. Thomas, Springfield, Ill.

TURNBULL, P. C. B., KRAMER, J. M., JØRGENSEN, K., GILBERT, R. J., & MELLING, J. (1979). 'Properties and production characteristics of vomiting, diarrheal and necrotizing toxins of *Bacillus cereus*.' *Am. J. Clin. Nut. 32*: 219.

WATSON, D. W. & KIM, Y. B. (1970). 'Erythrogenic toxins.' In: *Bacterial Toxins* Vol. III p. 173. Edited by T. C. Montie, S. Kadis, and S. J. Ajl. Academic Press.

6 Cell-associated toxins

In this chapter we will discuss bacterial toxins that, unlike the toxins covered throughout the rest of this book, are distinct cellular components and are not released into the surrounding medium in any quantity except upon death and lysis of the bacteria. These cell-associated toxins represent a small, heterogeneous group within a wide range of bacterial surface components that are known to contribute to pathogenesis and are termed 'agressins' (Smith 1977).

Endotoxins

Endotoxins are part of the outer membrane of Gram-negative bacteria. It has been known for many years that the cells (alive or dead) or cell extracts of a wide variety of Gram-negative bacteria are toxic to man and animals. The literature on this subject is vast, sometimes confusing and often controversial; here we can give no more than a brief outline. Some of the diseases in which endotoxin may play an important role include typhoid fever, tularaemia, plague, and brucellosis, and a variety of hospital-acquired infections caused by opportunistic Gram-negative pathogens which include *Escherichia coli, Proteus, Pseudomonas aeruginosa, Enterobacter, Serratia,* and *Klebsiella.* In addition, endotoxin has been intensively studied as a possible causative agent of shock arising from post-operative sepsis or other forms of traumatic injury in which the normal flora of the gut is regarded by some as the source of endotoxin.

The toxins we have considered so far have been protein (or at least part protein) in nature but, in contrast, endotoxin is a complex lipopolysaccharide. It is also much more heat-stable than protein toxins and much less easily toxoided. In addition to lethality, endotoxin displays a bewildering array of biological effects, the analysis of which has attracted enormous attention and generated a voluminous literature.

Location in cell envelope The complex nature of the multi-layered Gram-negative bacterial envelope is shown in Fig. 15. The outer membrane is composed of a bimolecular leaflet arrangement as are other membranes but has a different

Figure 15 Location and chemical structure of the lipopolysaccharide chain of *Salmonella typhimurium.* The abbreviations used are: 2-Ac-Abe: 2-D-acetyl abequose; Gal: galactose; Glc: glucose; Man: mannose; Rha: rhamnose; Hep: 1-glycero-D-man-noheptose; GlcNAcp: N-acetyl glucosamine; KDO: 2-keto-3-deoxyoctonate; p: pyranose, P: phosphate; FA: long chain fatty acids such as B-hydroxymyristic, myristic, palmitic, and lauric acid; GN: glucosamine.

(Composition of core and side chain polysaccharides from Luderitz, O., Westphal, O., Staub, A.M., and Nikaido, H., In 'Microbial Toxins' (Ed. by G. Weinbaum, S. Kadis, and S.Ail), **IV**, 127, Academic Press, 1971.)

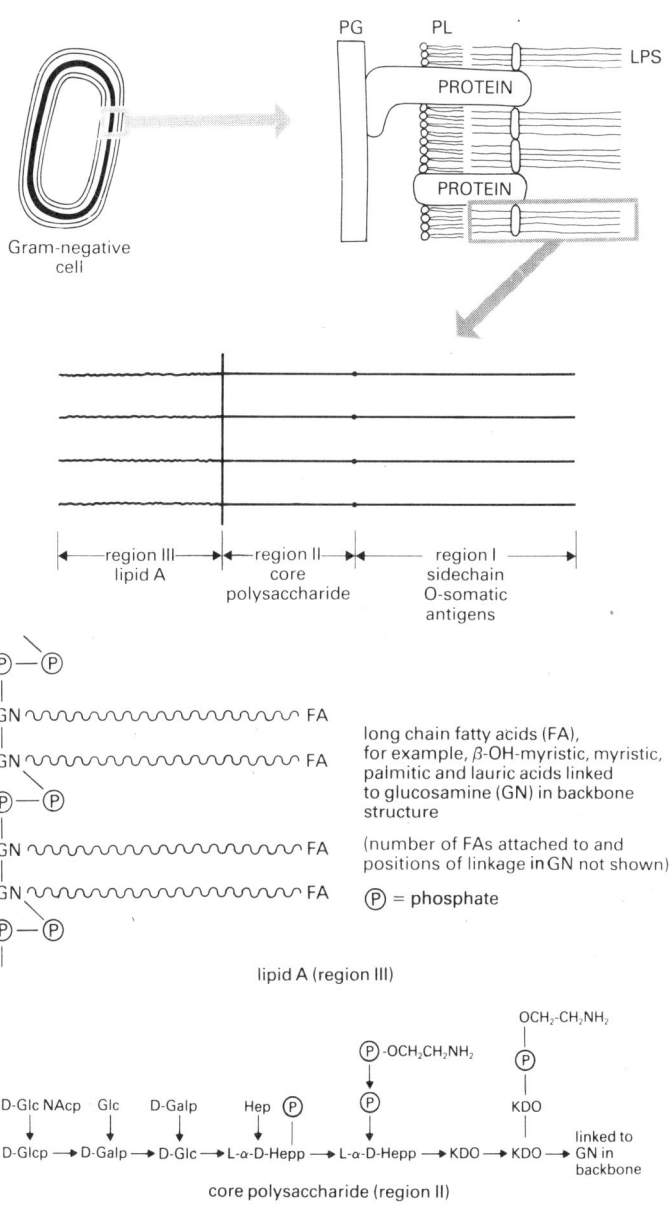

Gram-negative cell

PG PL

PROTEIN

PROTEIN

LPS

region III
lipid A

region II
core
polysaccharide

region I
sidechain
O-somatic
antigens

long chain fatty acids (FA),
for example, β-OH-myristic, myristic,
palmitic and lauric acids linked
to glucosamine (GN) in backbone
structure

(number of FAs attached to and
positions of linkage in GN not shown)

(P) = phosphate

lipid A (region III)

D-Glc NAcp   Glc   D-Galp   Hep (P)   (P)-OCH₂CH₂NH₂   OCH₂-CH₂NH₂

D-Glcp → D-Galp → D-Glc → L-α-D-Hepp → L-α-D-Hepp → KDO → KDO → GN in backbone

core polysaccharide (region II)

2-Ac-Abep   D-Glcp   2-Ac-Abep   linked to
D-Manp → L-Rhap → D-Galp   D-Manp → L-Rhap → D-Galp → D-Glcp in region II
                              7

O-specific chains (regions I)

Figure 15

composition from the cytoplasmic membrane. The lipopolysaccharide (LPS) is unique in nature, only found in Gram-negative bacteria, and is, or contains within it, what we designate endotoxin. Immunoelectron microscopy indicates that LPS exists in the outer leaflet of the membrane and extends outward up to 300 nm. Thus it is evident that the term endotoxin is a misnomer which derives from the era when toxins were considered to be either exotoxins, which were synthesized and secreted by the viable organism, or endotoxins, which were intracellular and released only upon lysis; but, Fig. 15 shows that endotoxin is *on* rather than *in* cells. Moreover, extraction with EDTA shows that approximately 50 per cent of LPS is held non-covalently linked in the membrane. Extraction with a variety of different solvents yields material which is highly heterogenous and of apparent molecular weight 1 to 20×10^6. However, treatment with pyridine or addition of detergents reduces the polydispersity. The endotoxic glycolipid from the rough mutant of *Salmonella minnesota*, R 595, has a molecular weight of 5900 for the basic unit, from which complex aggregate structures are derived.

Structure Lipopolysaccharide consists of three regions: polysaccharide side chains, core polysaccharide, and lipid A, which consists of a glucosamine phosphate backbone to which long chain fatty acids are linked (Fig. 15). The relationship of this type of molecule to the outer membrane is also shown in Fig. 15. The long chain fatty acids interdigitate between the phospholipids in the outer leaflet and may also be linked (or interact) with lipoproteins, which in turn may or may not be covalently anchored to the rigid peptidoglycan. The polysaccharide side chains project outwards.

This structure is not invariant. For example, many organisms when first isolated give rise to colonies with a smooth appearance on agar but on sub-culture produce colonies with a rough appearance. In general, 'smooth' strains of pathogenic species are more virulent than rough strains. This $S \rightarrow R$ conversion is accompanied by a loss of Region I side chains, which contain the deoxy- and dideoxy-sugars found in these LPS complexes. In addition to these somewhat drastic changes involving loss of side chains, it is possible to induce major compositional changes by manipulating the growth rate of these organisms in a chemostat. Thus the LPS of *Salmonella enteriditis*, when grown with a mean generation time of 20 min is nearly totally deficient in tyvelose (a dideoxysugar), possesses 85 per cent of the galactose and 150 per cent of the glucose contents of LPS obtained when the generation time is 50 min. These genotypic S organisms exhibit an R-phenotype in terms of their vastly reduced O-agglutinability (see below); such observations are potentially very important in the context of the *in vivo* phenotype and pathogenicity, since it is well known that the growth rate of *Salmonella typhimurium* in mice is 10–20 times lower than *in vitro*.

Structure; immunochemistry; seroclassification Before looking at the biological properties of LPS we feel a short digression on the immunochemistry of LPS is warranted. The extent to which lipid A is common between different genera is uncertain, but it is not likely to vary tremendously. The core polysaccharide structure is the same or very similar within groups of the Enterobacteriacae: thus polysaccharides from salmonellae are similar to each other, but differ from those of *E. coli* strains. However, within a group such as the salmonellae, there is a wide variation in the composition and detailed structures of the side chains, a fact which is exploited in the Kauffman-White scheme for classifying salmonellae.

The side chains carry the O-somatic antigen specificities of which there are far more than can readily be accounted for on the basis of the known number of sugars involved in the basic repeating units. However, the general principles governing the relationship between the various chemotypes and serotypes are now well understood; the multiplicity of antibody specificities evoked may be explained in terms of antibodies which can recognize different aspects of one three-dimensional structure.

Structure; biological properties The diversity and range of biological properties associated with endotoxin and the structural correlates of such activities is quite bewildering. Most people now accept that Lipid A is the primary toxiphore, but that the polysaccharide plays an important part in conferring solubility upon, and optimizing the size of micellar aggregates of LPS, hence affecting biological activity. However, the immune status of the test animal may affect toxicity: as normal animals produce antibodies to the antigenic determinants on the surface of normal gut organisms (including O-somatic antigens), the biological effects of endotoxin may be mediated by hypersensitivity mechanisms.

The most powerful evidence that lipid A is the primary toxiphore comes from studies on smooth and rough mutants whose biosynthetic capabilities are blocked at various points. This established that neither the O-side chains, nor the core polysaccharide are necessary for endotoxicity. A preparation of LPS containing only lipid A and 2-keto-3-deoxyoctanoate (KDO), designated Re (R, rough; e, one of a series of antigens designated a–e derived from certain rough mutant strains) possesses the same toxicity as LPS from S-strains. Removal of the KDO to yield free lipid reduces toxicity, probably by lowering the solubility of these preparations, but KDO is non-essential for toxicity: chemical modification of KDO does not impair biological activity of Re LPS. Moreover, pure lipid A can be made toxic by complexing it to a hydrophilic carrier like bovine serum albumin.

In the ensuing paragraphs we shall briefly review the biological properties of endotoxin, concentrating on those effects which might play an important role in Gram-negative bacterial infections: abortion, pyrogenicity and tolerance, Schwartzman phenomenon, hypotension and shock, and lethality.

Abortion The pregnant ungulate is susceptible to infection by *Brucella abortus*. This infection is marked by two dominant features: the localization and massive growth of the causative organism in the placental tissues and abortion of a usually dead foetus. The first phenomenon was shown by Pearce, Smith, Keppie and co-workers to be due to a predilection of *B. abortus* for erythritol, which is present in the susceptible tissues. The abortifacient is almost certainly endotoxin since injection of endotoxin preparations into pregnant guinea pigs, rabbits and rats (both by intravenous and intraperitoneal routes) induces abortion in nearly every case.

Pyrogenicity and tolerance In this section we shall discuss the biological mechanisms responsible for the production and release of endogenous pyrogen and the induction of a state of tolerance to this effect. We can then better appreciate the significance of some superb experiments carried out on human volunteers by Greisman and colleagues in an attempt to evaluate the potential role of endotoxin in the production of the febrile response associated with Gram-negative bacteraemias such as typhoid and tularaemia.

Pyrogenicity and tolerance have been studied extensively in rabbits and man: these two species exhibit on a weight basis a comparable degree of sensitivity to endotoxin. The minimum pyrogenic dose for man is $1-5$ ng/kg and this induces within $90-120$ min a monophasic febrile response of about 4 h duration. In the rabbit the response is biphasic: an initial rise in temperature occurs 15 min after injection and peaks by about 90 min; larger doses induce a second response similar to that seen in humans. The effects induced in man are dependent on the route of administration. For example, intradermal injection of small quantities $(0.1-1.0$ ng) induces, by 3 h, a gross inflammatory response, characterized by an infiltration of predominantly mononuclear cells. Increasing the concentration of endotoxin by about 100-fold results in an inflammatory response which is predominantly polymorphonuclear. Repeated intradermal injection of endotoxin over a period of a week does not induce a state of tolerance (defined and discussed below) but a persistence of the inflammatory response with infiltration of lymphocytes and macrophages.

When similar amounts of endotoxin are administered intravenously, however, a febrile response is evoked together with subjective toxic responses such as chills, rigor, headache, muscle pain, loss of appetite, nausea, and sometimes vomiting. Repeated daily injections in man induce a state of tolerance—that is, reduced febrile and subjective toxic responses; in rabbits the second but not the first febrile peak disappears. This state of tolerance is not absolute because the toxic manifestations of endotoxin can be elicited again by increasing the dose. Moreover, tolerance in this context is not to be confused with 'immunological tolerance', which is an inducible state of immunological unresponsiveness to an antigen; that is, a state in which an immune response is not elicited to an antigenic stimulus.

The overall picture of the biological mechanisms involved in fever production is fairly clear, though not the details of endotoxin/cell interactions responsible for the various aspect of the complex system. Anatomically, intact connections are required between the anterior hypothalamus and the cervical cord for both normal thermoregulation and the action of endotoxin. Endotoxin directly affects the central nervous system when injected into the brain: the toxin remains localized and the onset of effects is rapid and the outcome fatal. It appears that an intact nervous system is not important in the initiation of endotoxin-mediated effects, but has a profound influence in the subsequent course of events. The delay between the injection of endotoxin (by all other routes) and the onset of fever was originally interpreted to mean that endotoxin was acting indirectly on the hypothalamus by stimulating production of an endogenous pyrogen. Several observations seemed to point to the importance of circulating granulocytes as the tissue from which such endogenous pyrogen(s) (protein(s) of molecular weight $10-20\,000$) were released. Injections of large doses of endotoxin to rabbits induce a depression in the numbers of circulating white cells (leucopaenia). This is caused by endotoxin-induced sticking of leucocytes in capillaries and is followed by a progressive rise in the number of circulating white cells (leucocytosis) owing to release of immature granulocytes from the bone marrow, and, onset of fever. Incubation of leucocytes with endotoxin *in vitro* causes inactivation of endotoxin and release of pyrogen, which can also be extracted from such cells. These and other supporting observations focused attention for many years on circulating leucocytes as the major source of endogenous pyrogen. While these cells are still regarded as a source of pyrogen, the following evidence suggests that hepatic Kupffer cells (phagocytic cells which line the sinusoids of the liver) are the principal source of endogenous pyrogen.

Isolated Kupffer cells from rabbits, just like blood leucocytes, can be stimulated by endotoxin to release endogenous pyrogen, but only Kupffer cells and not blood leucocytes from endotoxin-tolerant animals are refractory to endotoxin-mediated release of pyrogen. Moreover, intravenously injected endotoxin is mainly sequestered by hepatic Kupffer cells in rabbits, and studies involving direct injection of endotoxin into the liver *via* the hepatic portal vein show that the liver is primarily responsible for release of endogenous pyrogen during the second, but not the first febrile phase, and refractoriness to this effect.

There is little doubt about the involvement of endogenous pyrogen. It can be produced *in vitro* and its effects demonstrated *in vivo*. It can be stimulated *in vivo* and transferred to another animal, which will undergo a febrile response. However, in recent years it has become clear that prostaglandins may be involved as the terminal mediators of the febrile response. Direct injection of prostaglandin into the brain causes fever and injection of endotoxin into the brain results in synthesis or release of prostaglandin and evokes fever. Inhibitors of prostaglandin synthesis or release (for example, aspirin or indomethacin) suppress the febrile response. Prostaglandin levels are elevated in the plasma of endotoxin-shocked dogs. It is also known that prostaglandins are produced in many different tissues.

Thus endotoxin could cause fever by a direct effect on the thermoregulatory centres: the question of a direct mode of action in addition to an induced mediator mechanism must be considered in all aspects of endotoxin activity. The first febrile peak observed in animals may be due to the direct action of endotoxin. Additionally, endotoxin is *known* to induce production of endogenous pyrogen. This may act on the hypothalamus directly or, *via* prostaglandins, synthesized or released locally in brain tissue after the arrival of endogenous pyrogen, or in other extra-neural tissues.

The mechanism of tolerance is complex and here we give in outline the analysis and the model developed by Greisman and Hornick. In both rabbit and man, continuous intravenous infusion or closely spaced injections of low levels of endotoxin induces a tolerant state within hours which is readily overcome by increasing the rate of infusion or size of subsequent injections. The speed of induction of tolerance, its lack of specificity between differing endotoxins, its non-transferability with serum, its non-association with increasing levels of antibody in normal animals, its induction in splenectomized animals (which are suppressed in their ability to synthesize antibody to endotoxin), an increase in the rate of clearance of endotoxin by the reticuloendothelial system (RES) but no demonstrable increase in ability of plasma or liver homogenates to inactivate endotoxin, all argue strongly in favour of a direct endotoxin-cell interaction which inhibits synthesis and/or release of endogenous pyrogen. During this state both man and rabbit are responsive to preformed pyrogen.

It is now clear, however, that a second, demonstrably different phase of tolerance is induced in both man and rabbit after 3–4 days. In particular, it is transferable with serum, suggesting a role for antibody against either O-specific side chain determinants or the less specific core-specific antibodies, depending on whether the inducing preparation was derived from smooth or rough strains of organisms. The mechanism of antibody-mediated tolerance is probably to prevent release of pyrogen. Some workers have failed to recognize the existence of the two types of tolerance mechanism and this has led to considerable confusion in the past.

The final point we wish to deal with relates to the phagocytic role of the RES in tolerance. It was thought that tolerance was due only to the enhanced rate of clearance of endotoxin by the RES, of which hepatic Kupffer cells constitute such an important segment. On this basis it was thought that endotoxin was more quickly diverted by an activated RES from other primary target sites (for example, circulating granulocytes). Earlier experiments which seemed to confirm this hypothesis consisted of blockading the RES (that is, saturating the phagocytic activity of these cells with suitable agents), as a result of which the responsiveness of the tolerant animal returned to levels comparable with that of normal animals. This theory predicts that direct introduction of endotoxin into Kupffer cells *via* the hepatic portal vein, thereby effectively by-passing circulating granulocytes, should result in no pyrogenic response in a non-tolerant animal. However, there is a response comparable with that induced using other routes.

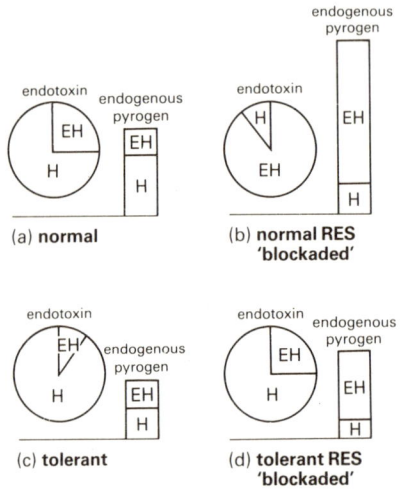

(a) normal   (b) normal RES 'blockaded'

(c) tolerant   (d) tolerant RES 'blockaded'

Figure 16 Endotoxin, tolerance, and RES system. The circle segments denote the relative proportions of endotoxin removed from circulation by the Kupffer cells and extra-hepatic tissues; the columns denote the relative proportions of endogenous pyrogen released from these tissues. Increase in release of pyrogen in (b) as compared with (a) arises because the RES is blockaded and hence less endotoxin is phagocytosed (and detoxified) in the liver and therefore diverted to extra-hepatic sites. Evidence points to the fact that early non-antibody mediated tolerance arises from an increased rate of clearance of endotoxin by the liver (i.e. enhanced phagocytosis) *and* a concomitant decrease in ability to synthesize/release endogenous pyrogen in response to phagocytosis (c). Blockade of the RES in the tolerant animal (d) means that less endotoxin is phagocytosed by the liver than in (c) and more is diverted to the extra-hepatic tissues to produce a pyrogen releasing effect whose total is similar to that described in (a) but whose internal distribution is different. The level at which antibody acts in late tolerance is probably by interfering with some RES/endotoxin-receptor mechanism.

RES: reticuloendothelial system (important branch of which is Kupffer cells in the liver); H: hepatic; EH: extra-hepatic.

(After Greisman, S.E. and Hornick, R.B., (1973), *J. Inf. Dis. Suppl.*, **28**, 257.)

The picture, based on the work of Greisman and Wolff (summarized in Fig. 16), becomes clearer when one includes for comparison the effect of blockading the RES in normal as well as tolerant animals. Blockading the tolerant animal restores a total responsiveness which is comparable with that of the normal animal but significantly lower than the blockaded normal animal. Thus blockading the RES makes both normal *and* tolerant animals hyper-reactive to endotoxin but does *not* abolish the striking differences in reactivity between comparable normal and tolerant animals. This is because although accelerated uptake of endotoxin into Kupffer phagocytic cells is demonstrable in both the non-antibody and antibody-mediated phases of tolerance, the refractory state is accompanied by a decreased ability of Kupffer cells *to release* endogenous pyrogen. Thus accelerated clearance into Kupffer cells is only an ancillary mechanism whose importance lies in the rate at which endotoxin is phagocytozed by cells which are refractory to release of endogenous pyrogen and hence kept away from susceptible extra-hepatic cells.

Greisman and his colleagues have also tackled the questions of the microbial determinants of the sustained pyrexia so characteristic of typhoid and tularaemia. They produced clinical typhoid and tularaemia in human volunteers, who developed a hyper-reactivity to the pyrogenic and subjective toxic activities of endotoxin. Within this hyper-reactive framework, tolerance was still inducible either by continuous infusion or by daily injections of endotoxin: hyper-elevated temperatures dropped and endotoxin was rapidly cleared from the blood. Tolerance mechanisms induced before experimental infection could also be demonstrated during illness. Such observations on the ability of man to acquire tolerance during typhoidal and tularaemic illness, and the inability to mitigate these illnesses by deliberate induction of tolerance, would suggest that circulating endotoxin does not constitute the major cause of the sustained pyrexia and toxaemia during these illnesses. A similar situation pertains in human brucellosis. Does this mean then that endotoxin plays no role in these diseases?

It is exceedingly difficult to demonstrate circulating endogenous pyrogen in humans undergoing a febrile response. Endotoxin is certainly made because the organisms concerned multiply to high levels, and it must be released, at least during the terminal stages, since tolerance to endotoxin is demonstrable during convalescence. Thus either endotoxin plays no role in fever or only very small quantities of endotoxin are required to initiate fever under the conditions of an infection *in vivo*.

Greisman and co-workers make the suggestion that endotoxin could still be responsible for the systemic effects seen in typhoid and tularaemia by virtue of its ability to generate pyrogen within a local inflammatory situation. This is possible because systemic tolerance in man induced by intravenous injection does not induce tolerance to local dermal reactivity (see above). On the contrary, local effects are enhanced. They point out that 'this concept would be consonant with the inability to mitigate this illness' (typhoid fever) 'by deliberate induction of systemic tolerance to intravenously-injected endotoxin.'

Schwartzman reaction This can take two forms. The local Schwartzman reaction occurs when an intradermal priming injection of endotoxin is followed by an intravenous injection some hours later; the second injection elicits a local skin necrosis. The generalized Schwartzman reaction (GSR) is evoked by giving an intravenous priming injection followed 24 h later by another intravenous injection of endotoxin. GSR has been widely studied as a biological phenomenon but also

Bacterial Toxins

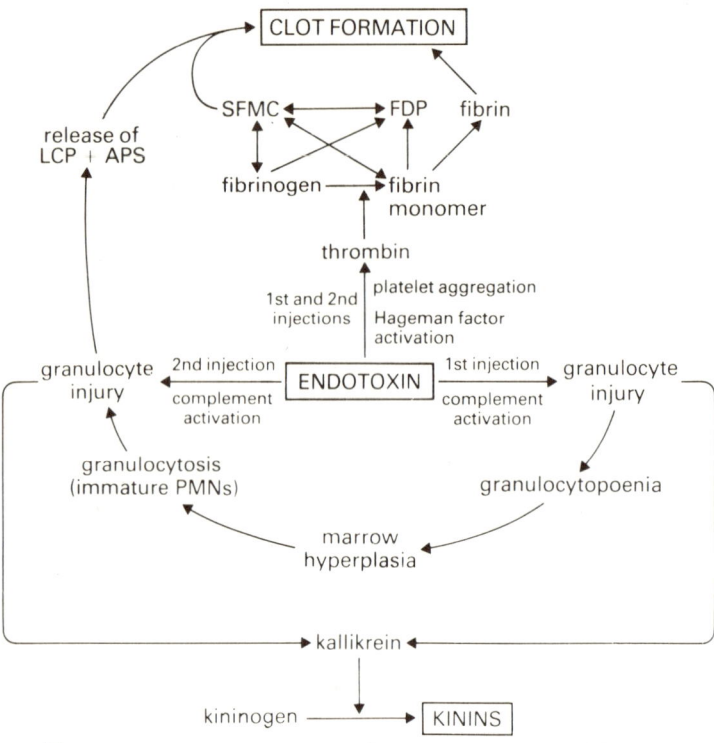

Figure 17 Endotoxin induced generalized Schwartzman reaction (GSR) and elevated kinin levels. The feature around which these two biological phenomena have been centred is the effect of endotoxin on the number and nature of circulating granulocytes. One injection induces injury to, followed by a drop in numbers of, granulocytes; some 24 h later, huge numbers of immature cells are released into the circulation from bone marrow. The first injection also triggers formation of SFMC and some fibrin. The second injection given to evoke the GSR at the peak of granulocytosis results in release (this time in large quantities) of LCP and APS which interact with SFMC to form clots which may either be fibrin (arising from dissociation of SFMC) or hetero-complexes with SFMC itself; this later para-coagulation phenomenon can be reproduced by a variety of charged polymers. The elevation of kinin levels is an exceedingly complex process involving many mechanisms sensitive to endotoxin-triggering. Here we show only how kallikrein is released from endotoxin-injured cells leading to an activation of kininogen to form kinin (an oligopeptide), which may be responsible for inducing hypotension in endotoxin-shocked primates. It has been postulated that species-specific variations in response to endotoxin could in part reflect the known differences in the kinin-inducing capacity of granulocytes of different species.

LCP: lysosomal cationic proteins; SFMC: soluble fibrin-monomer-complexes; APS: acidic polysaccharide; GSR: generalized Schwartzman reaction; FDP: fibrin degradation products.

(After 1, Horn, R. G., and 2, Miller, R. L., Reichgott, M. J., and Melmon, K. L., (1973), *J. Inf. Dis. Suppl.* **128**, **126** and **136** respectively.)

because its characteristic features, intravascular coagulation together with shock, are among the most serious complications that can arise with Gram-negative bacterial infections.

GSR is characterized primarily by the development of intravascular clotting, in particular glomerular capillary thrombosis, and secondarily by renal cortical necrosis. The mechanisms involved are highly complex and not completely understood, hence no attempt will be made to deal with this in detail. Only a summary will be given of how endotoxin might trigger the complex process of clotting in the genesis of GSR. Experimental evidence argues against RES blockade and impaired fibrinolysis but in favour of a granulocyte-mediated enhancement of clotting. Following injection of endotoxin, there is depression in the numbers of circulating granulocytes followed by a marked increase in the numbers of granulocytes from the bone marrow. The new cells are immature, contain a high proportion of granules rich in highly-charged proteins, and their numbers peak between 12–14 h after the first injection. In addition, a transient low-grade intravascular coagulation occurs which may be partly responsible for the reduction in circulating granulocytes. Maximal sensitivity to clotting exists when the second injection is given about 24 h after the first, when numbers of circulating granulocytes are at their peak. Accordingly, treatments (nitrogen mustard, for example) which depress the numbers of granulocytes, diminish sensitivity to GSR. Moreover, GSR effects can be induced instantaneously in the lungs by a single injection of endotoxin (if given intravenously) and in the kidney (if given *via* the aorta) in normal or in severly granulocytopoenic rabbits; however, for this to happen, the endotoxin must be accompanied by polymorphonuclear neutrophils (PMNs), granules from PMNs or soluble extracts of granules.

What role can be ascribed to the granulocyte in GSR? An attractive scheme has been developed (Fig. 17) which incorporates several features. First it focuses attention on the granulocytosis which occurs after initial granulocytopoenia. Second, it highlights the diversity of endotoxin biological activity, which in this clot-producing scheme involves activation of the complement system, platelet aggregation, and activation of Hageman (XII) factor. Third, the action of endotoxin is seen to be basically the same following each injection, with the important additional input after the second injection of the products of granulocyte damage on a much larger scale than after the priming injection. The mechanism of clot-formation resides in the para-coagulation phenomena giving rise to various forms of soluble fibrin, including soluble fibrin monomer complex (SFMC), as shown in Fig. 17. The production of a dynamic state (leading to low quantities of fibrin which are presumably dealt with by the plasmin and RES systems) is possible because of endotoxin activation of the clot-forming cascade in the first instance. However, the administration of the provoking dose of endotoxin results in release from granulocytes of charged proteins which can either dissociate SFMC, allowing fibrin to spontaneously aggregate to form fibrin clots, or form insoluble complexes with SFMC itself. There is evidence that synthetic charged polymers will, along with endotoxin, cause intravascular coagulation.

Hypotension and shock Before discussing the role of endotoxin in producing this complex syndrome we must first define shock. Primary or neurogenic shock is a state whose rapid onset is caused by damage to the neurological system with loss of vital motor function. Secondary shock encompasses effects which are secondary to some other primary injury or trauma. There are four states in the development of this clinical condition. The *initial stage*, when the volume of circulating blood decreases, but insufficiently to cause serious symptoms. This is followed by a *compensatory stage*, when blood volume is further reduced and the body begins to compensate. Blood pressure is maintained by vasoconstriction, which selectively diverts blood from skin (hence the blanched appearance) and kidney, and depletes main reservoirs such as the spleen; blood supply to the central nervous system and myocardium is maintained. The third or *progressive stage* is one in which the unfavourable changes (falling blood pressure, increasing vasoconstriction, accelerated heart rate, decreased pulse pressure, deficient urine excretion and so on) increase and the compensatory mechanisms fail to compensate. This leads to the fourth or *irreversible stage*, when treatment, including blood transfusion, is hopeless. Blood remains pooled in peripheral beds with no significant flow rate and hence poor perfusion of tissues.

This clinical state is often seen in infectious disease. There are many routes to this common clinical terminus and the specificity of disease lies in the inductive mechanism responsible for decreased blood flow and pressure. This could arise from any direct cardiotoxic action which would affect cardiac output. Alternatively, there are various indirect means whereby the haemodynamic situation could be impaired. Clearly, any mechanism which affects the venous return to the 'right heart' will affect the ability of the 'left heart' to pump sufficient blood to the tissues. Endotoxin could activate localized generation of histamine or systemic generation of kinins—hypotensive agents which act by increasing capillary permeability and by vasodilatation—thus causing leakage of blood into extravascular spaces. Blocking mechanisms such as in GSR could also operate. Vasoconstrictors such as the catecholamines affect renal blood flow, and histamine also contracts the smooth muscle of the hepatic vein. One must also consider the effect on the autonomic nervous system, which is important in controlling circulation: endotoxins may act directly or indirectly on key centres of the central nervous system. Here the arguments become somewhat circular. Does such neural activity initiate some of the responses already described or merely augment or exacerbate them?

There is no doubt that injection of endotoxin will induce a shock-like syndrome and, depending on the dose, kill the animal. There are, however, two main questions which have been intensively studied and often hotly debated over several decades. First, what are the precise mechanisms involved in endotoxaemia? Second, what role, if any, does endotoxin play in non-septic shock—that is, shock arising from injury and not overt bacterial infection?

The pathophysiology of endotoxaemia is a complex and confused field. Experimental studies have centred on the dog and sub-human primates, which exhibit marked differences in their response to endotoxin (Table 9). Not surprisingly, monkeys resemble man more than do dogs—another important reminder to the student concerning the use of experimental models. The following brief discussion, which is restricted to these two species, serves as an introduction to how this complex problem has been approached.

The most studied aspect in both species is the initial drop in blood pressure. In the dog there is an explosive release of vasoactive agents, about whose precise role there is still disagreement. We shall consider only histamine and the catecholamines although others are also involved.

Histamine is released after injection of endotoxin either by direct action on histamine-releasing cells or *via* the production of anaphylotoxin due to endotoxin

Table 9 Responses of the dog and monkey to endotoxin

	Parameter	Dog	Monkey
Similar	cardiac output	decrease	decrease
	direct cardiotoxic action	none	none
	venous return	decrease	decrease
	white cell count	decrease	decrease
Different	systemic arterial blood pressure	rapid drop[1]	gradual decline[2]
	total peripheral resistance	decrease	little change
	portal vein pressure	increase[1]	little change[2]
	hepatosplanchnic congestion	extensive	negligible
	visceral lesions	extensive	absent
	haematocrit	increase[1]	little change[2]
	haemolysis	present	absent
	catecholamine release	early, marked	late

1, 2 These changes reproducible by injecting histamine. Although there are differences between species, the effect of endotoxin and histamine is similar within each species. After L. B. Hinshaw (1971).

activation of the complement system. This could at least partly explain the effects of endotoxin injection in the dog, all of which are reproducible by injecting histamine. Moreover, some workers have demonstrated that antihistamines can prevent some of these effects. However, although histamine-induced haemodynamic alterations are so similar to those of endotoxin, not all experimental evidence supports the view, outlined above, implicating histamine release as the primary endotoxin-mediated event. For example, there are differences in response to endotoxin and 48/80 (a potent histamine releaser), and some experiments have failed to demonstrate increased levels of circulating histamine in dogs given a *sub-lethal* injection of endotoxin. Moreover, the haemodynamic effects of histamine are not specific and can also be produced by acetyl choline. It has been suggested that the discrepancies between endotoxin and 48/80 could be caused by different rates of histamine release from various storage sites, the elaboration of vasoactive agents other than histamine, and the peculiar direct effects of each agent.

The role of catecholamines is also controversial. They are probably released in the dog as part of the homeostatic response to the fall in arterial blood pressure, rather than in direct response to endotoxin. Baroreceptors are absent from the mesenteric circulation and hence protective responses are directed towards the needs of other organs, often at the expense of the gut. Thus catecholamines, released from the adrenals, close down the peripheral blood supply. Gut mucosal arterioles are particularly sensitive to circulating catecholamines whereas the submucosal arteriovenous shunts are not (see Fig. 18). Thus gut mucosa becomes deprived of its blood supply and becomes ischaemic. In addition, some believe that direct endotoxin-induced hyperactivity of the sympathetic nervous system causes damage by local release of the catecholamine norepinephrine; this would also induce gut stasis, which becomes progressively more dangerous under conditions of impaired blood supply.

Mesenteric circulation is necessary for the maintenance of bowel functions, including digestion, secretion, absorption; motility; rapid mucosal cell replacement; containment of tissue-destructive enzymes, noxious bacteria and/or their products; and maintenance of structural integrity. Visceral ischaemia may interfere with any or all of these functions and may progress from mild to disastrous, depending on the extent, rate of onset, and site of the ischaemic process and the

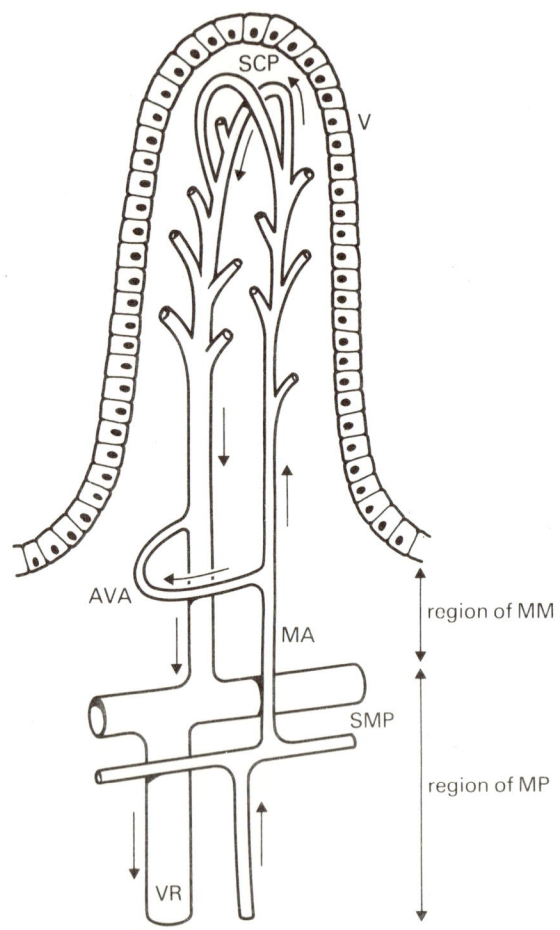

Figure 18 Schematic representation of microcirculation of gut.

SCP: surface capillary plexus; AVA: arteriovenous anastamosis (shunt); MA: mucosal artery; SMP: submucosal vascular plexus; VR: venous return; MM: muscularis mucosae; MP: muscularis propria; V: villus.
(After Edwards, A. J., (1975), *Medicine* **19**, 909.)

species affected. In the dog, the gut becomes congested, haemorrhagic and oedematous, because of the lack of valves in the portal system and hence the backflow of blood into the low pressure ischaemic areas. Fine's theory is that this is the major pathological change, at least in the dog. Damage allows absorption of more endotoxin from the gut, which because of impaired RES activity, particularly in the congested liver, is not inactivated but perpetuates this catastrophic cascade until the animal dies.

In the primate the decline in arterial blood pressure is more gradual; catecholamine levels rise much later in shock as compared with the dog. In addition there are also marked differences in the extent of hepatosplanchnic pooling and severity of lesions in the gut. The latter may become ischaemic without becoming necrotic as in the dog. The principal pathology is seen in the lung, which becomes congested and oedematous. The resulting impairment in oxygen uptake, allied to haemodynamic changes, causes generalized metabolic derangement.

While the precise details of the changes in lung function are not fully clear, the mechanism(s) responsible for the hypotension is almost certainly due to peripheral vasodilatation. Histamine probably plays a less significant role in the monkey than in the dog, as judged by the effects produced on histamine injection, suggesting the involvement of some other agent. Some have argued the case for bradykinin (one of a family of kinins; oligopeptides with vasodilatory properties) as the agent responsible for this phenomenon. It has not been possible to dissociate early cardiovascular failure from elevated kinin production, but equally the two have never been unequivocally causally related. There is a multiplicity of mechanisms whereby endotoxin can enhance circulating kinin levels *in vivo* (only one is shown in Fig. 17). It may be that the species variability in endotoxin-induced shock could reflect the nature of kinin-generating enzymes released from circulating leucocytes as a result of interaction with the lipid moeity of LPS. Certainly human cells release a rapidly acting kininogenase which activates kininogen to form kinin. Other studies show that catecholamines are released much later in shock. In conclusion, the basis of species-variation and in particular which mechanism (the sympathoadrenal or kinin systems) is initially activated in endotoxin-induced shock are unknown.

Endotoxaemia: septic and non-septic shock Although the precise mechanisms of endotoxaemia are still uncertain, the foregoing section at least suggests that it is reasonable to attribute a state of shock in patients suffering from Gram-negative infections to circulating endotoxin. Fine and his colleagues demonstrated endotoxin in the circulation of some patients with both septic and non-septic disorders. However, since circulating endotoxin is not always detectable, even by the most sensitive tests, they looked for, and demonstrated, endotoxin in *post-mortem* tissue extracts in 20 out of 35 randomly selected patients. Attention was focused on the liver because animals dying of endotoxic shock contain relatively high levels of endotoxin in the liver (and spleen) immediately after death. There was a good correlation between endotoxin in the liver and gastrointestinal bleeding, haemorrhagic ulceration of the gastrointestinal mucosa, acute pulmonary pathology and major injury to the liver, a picture often associated with experimental endotoxaemia.

The demonstration of endotoxin in the tissues of patients without a septic focus supports the view developed by Fine over several decades that clinical shock in patients suffering from trauma is precipitated by endotoxin from the intestinal flora. In such a situation it is physical loss of blood (as in haemorrhagic shock) which gives rise to lowered blood pressure, whereas in experimental endotoxaemia it is the evocation of a complex mechanism involving release of pharmacologically active compounds which precipitates the fatal cascade. In both cases, pathological changes increase absorption of endotoxin (derived from intestinal flora) and decrease the ability of the RES to detoxify it.

This view seemed to be supported by experiments in rabbits in which the nature of the intestinal flora was manipulated by prior antibiotic treatment. After massive injury induced by an intravenous injection of endotoxin (100 μg/kg), rabbits with a normal flora showed a high level of endotoxin in plasma, liver, spleen, and lung at death or at 24 h post injection when surviving animals were killed. By comparison, rabbits pretreated with kanamycin injected into the intestine or rabbits with predominantly Gram-positive flora accumulated low levels in these tissues.

Two lines of evidence, however, conflict with Fine's views. His theory predicts that gnotobiotic animals should be resistant to shock; they are not, or at least this has never been convincingly and reproducibly demonstrated. This may be because a gnotobiotic diet is sterile but not necessarily endotoxin free. Moreover, germ-free animals may not have the same intestinal absorption characteristics as 'normal' animals. However, both clinical observations on patients and experiments on rabbits by Kass's group cast strong doubt at least on the *uniqueness* of endotoxin in inducing lethal shock. They used a rabbit skin test to detect endotoxin in the plasma of septic patients and showed that not every patient who died of septic shock had Gram-negative bacterial infections—some were associated with Gram-positive bacterial infections. Furthermore, although circulating endotoxin of intestinal origin could be demonstrated in rabbits in which hypotension is induced by controlled haemorrhage, the presence or absence of endotoxin was irrelevant to the ultimate fatal outcome in rabbits, and by extension, in humans. They claim that factors other than endotoxin are important.

It is difficult to reconcile such apparently contradictory results. Perhaps different methods used to induce experimental injury in rabbits affect the outcome, or factors other than endotoxin can also produce irreversible shock by virtue of their ability to stimulate the complement system, which can play a vital role in the genesis of lethal shock. In this respect, there are increasing reports that peptidoglycan of the Gram-positive cell wall possesses endotoxin-like properties (for example, it is pyrogenic and complement-activating) and this may well be the key to unlocking this problem.

Lethality Are additional mechanisms involved in endotoxin lethality? In view of the known diverse activities of endotoxin it would scarcely be surprising if lethality is the result of the integrated sum of all the many events (including some not covered in this section) which comprise the endotoxin pathophysiological cascade. However, more recent work points to the importance of endotoxin-lymphoid cell interaction in the terminal stages of lethality. Mice which are genetically resistant to the lethal effects of endotoxin were rendered sensitive by transfer of spleen cells from histocompatible endotoxin-sensitive mice. The mechanism and significance of this is uncertain but we know that endotoxin activates B-lymphocytes to release mediators of various immunological phenomena including the activation of macrophages. One such signal is prostaglandin(s), known to play a role in pyrogenicity.

Thus endotoxin death may be the result of the overstimulation of a variety of normal processes to an extent with which the body cannot cope.

Protection against lethal effects of endotoxin or bacteraemia with antibody Antibodies can be raised to structures on the core section of LPS as well as to 0-specific determinants on the side chains. GSR can be prevented by antiserum active against determinants present in rough LPS, with a significant cross-protection when heterologous LPS is used to provoke the GSR. Furthermore, McCabe and co-workers, in 1973, using mice immunized with *Salmonella minnesota* S218, a variety of chemically defined rough mutants (Ra60, Rb345, Rc5, Rd7, $Rd_2$3 and Re595) derived from this organism, and *Escherichia coli* 0 : 14 as a source of the Kunin common antigen (CA, common to a variety of enterobacteria), showed that animals passively or actively immunized against Re antigen resisted intravenous lethal challenge with *E. coli*, and *K. pneumoniae* better than with antibodies elicited by the other immunogenic stimuli. Later work points to the requirement of KDO (see Fig. 15) as being important because antibodies to lipid A are not protective.

The protective property of LPS is currently an active field of investigation which has been excellently summarized in a 1977 symposium on bacterial vaccines. An increasing number of organisms and hosts have been studied and the results, though not absolute, more than justify the pursuit of a broad spectrum immunogen effective against a range of Gram-negative organisms, particularly in view of the emergence of antibiotic resistance in several species. Moreover, the advantages of an immunoprophylactic approach are evident even in situations where the organism is sensitive to antibiotics, because of the problem of antibiotic-induced endotoxin release from dead organisms.

Endotoxin; coda We have not attempted to discuss every aspect of the biological activity of endotoxin but have concentrated on those aspects which are of potential importance in primary infectious disease or in secondary infections (or intoxication) consequent upon some other form of injury. It is obvious that to cause pathophysiological distress or death, an organism must have other attributes enabling it to gain access to sites where replication and release, from cells or cell walls of endotoxin can take place. Endotoxin is not in general a virulence attribute since it is possessed by avirulent strains of pathogens and by non-pathogens. However, even non-pathogens in the gut can and do cause endotoxaemia after alteration of gut permeability and absorption of toxin.

Finally, the Gram-negative bacterial cell wall, as mentioned already, is subject to considerable variations in both the composition of LPS and in the number and nature of the proteins found in the outer cell-membrane. Such phenotypic variation in LPS has rarely been examined in the context of pathogenicity but, as we shall see in the next section, the examination of cell-bound proteins of *Yersinia pestis* from organisms grown *in vivo* led to the discovery of a toxin lethal for mice and guinea pigs.

Toxins of *Yersinia pestis*

Plague is one of the most deadly diseases of man and has, over several thousands of years, claimed millions of lives. In the fourteenth century, 'the black death' wiped out a quarter of the population of Europe before spreading through the Middle East and Asia. Fortunately, however, the last sixty years or so have seen a drastic decrease in outbreaks of plague, though the threat of another epidemic is still with us.

The causative organism of plague, *Yersinia pestis*, is primarily a parasite of rodents in which it is endemic in many areas of the world. Only when man comes into close proximity with infected rodents do outbreaks of human plague occur. The disease is spread from rat to rat and from rat to man by fleas. Rodents in the terminal stages of infection with *Y. pestis* suffer massive bacteraemia and so when a flea sucks the blood of an infected animal it swallows large numbers of bacteria. When the rodent eventually dies, the flea leaves the corpse and awaits a new host. In the meantime, however, *Y. pestis* multiplies rapidly in the alimentary tract of the insect, often completely blocking the proventriculus. The flea becomes voraciously hungry and feeds on any suitable host, which sooner or later is man. However, because the flea's alimentary canal is blocked by bacteria it cannot feed efficiently and usually succeeds in imbibing blood only to regurgitate it, now contaminated with *Y. pestis*, back into the wound. During the next 2–8 days, organisms become localized and multiply in the regional lymph nodes, causing considerable swelling. These swellings, which are often in the inguinal region because the most common sites for flea-bites are the legs, are referred to as primary buboes; hence the name bubonic plague. Secondary buboes may develop, followed by necrosis of the lymphoid tissue and a progressive destruction of vascular integrity giving rise to haemorrhaging in many organs and tissues. These pathological changes are accompanied by prostration, high fever, delirium and high pulse rate, followed in the terminal stages of the disease by shock and death.

Little is known of the mechanism by which *Y. pestis* causes tissue damage and death, but the symptoms described above are indicative of a toxaemia. The principal features of human plague can be reproduced in guinea pigs and mice. Monkeys show shock-like signs only during the terminal period of 6–10 h, when they become quiet, lethargic, progressively weak, prostrate and hypothermic; for the previous 2–4 days infected animals are lively and vigorous. In the terminal stages blood pressure drops rapidly but there is no evidence of oligaemia caused by haemorrhage, or oedema suggesting that vascular collapse must be associated with a vasodilatory factor(s), resulting in pooling of blood. In this respect monkeys differ from humans and guinea pigs.

Evidence for the involvement of a toxin(s) was presented as long ago as 1928 by Dieudonne and Otto, who showed that foetuses of mothers dying from plague suffered extensive tissue damage but were free of detectable organisms. This was considerably strengthened in 1953 when McCrumb and his co-workers showed that antibiotics given 36–48 h after the onset of disease failed to save patients despite the fact that their blood and organs were sterile. These findings led to the search for, and recognition of, several antigens of *Y. pestis* possessing toxic activity. However, the severity of the disease for man has made it impossible to assess the role of these antigens in human plague, and our knowledge derives mainly from studies on mice, guinea pigs, and monkeys.

Plague endotoxin The symptoms of plague—high fever and vascular destruction—are characteristic of intoxication with endotoxin, but for many years isolation of endotoxin from *Y. pestis* eluded all investigators. Endotoxin was eventually isolated by Davies and shown to be toxic to a variety of experimental animals, albeit in very large quantities. However, improved methods of purification led eventually to the demonstration that endotoxin from *Y. pestis*, when injected into mice and guinea pigs, produces pathological lesions that closely resemble those caused by experimental infection; disruption of vascular integrity, leakage of plasma leading to haemoconcentration, and haemorrhaging in many organs, particularly the liver. However, the amounts of endotoxin needed to produce these lesions are much higher than the levels of cell-associated endotoxin encountered in the natural infection, and hence the importance of endotoxin alone in pathogenesis must be in doubt. Nevertheless, this does not preclude a role for endotoxin in conjunction with one or more other potentially toxic fractions from *Y. pestis*.

Plague murine toxin In 1910, Rowland isolated a toxin from *Y. pestis* by extraction with chloroform. This toxin, which he called Substance B, killed rats within 18 h. Later studies by Girard and other French workers showed the toxin to be cell-associated, but to resemble classical exotoxins in not possessing a lipoplysaccharide complex and in the ease with which it could be toxoided. Further purification of the toxin confirmed early observations that, although it is highly lethal for mice and rats, it is relatively non-toxic for other experimental animals such as guinea pigs, rabbits, dogs, and monkeys. For this reason the toxin has come to be known as plague murine toxin.

The toxin was first purified in 1958 and subsequently shown to be a protein of molecular weight 120 000 daltons. However, further work revealed the existence of a second toxic protein of molecular weight 240 000 daltons which is probably a dimer of the former toxin: both have an LD_{50} for mice of $0.5-1.0$ μg when injected intraperitoneally, and both are composed of seemingly identical $12-24000$ subunits.

The only detailed investigations into the pathology of animals intoxicated with preparations of murine toxin were carried out in the mid 1950s by Schar and his colleagues, who found that $16-24$ h after injection of toxin mice exhibited oedema and decrease in blood pressure resulting in shock. The most striking pathological lesions were in the liver, which was covered in small yellow necrotic patches. Microscopic examination revealed epithelial degeneration in both the liver and kidneys. Exactly similar lesions are observed in animals suffering from *Y. pestis* infection, suggesting that death due to murine toxin and natural infection is a consequence of peripheral vascular collapse. However, the toxic preparation almost certainly contained significant quantities of endotoxin, which could account for some of the pathological lesions described by Schar. Therefore, the ability of murine toxin to cause relevant pathology remains uncertain.

Despite this uncertainty, the observations of Schar that murine toxin apparently induces necrotic foci in the liver encouraged several workers in the USA to attempt to determine the mode of action of the toxin at the molecular level by investigating the effect of toxin on oxidative metabolism of mouse liver homogenates. The results of these studies were dramatic and perhaps unfortunate in that they diverted attention away from pathogenicity studies in animals. Ajl and his colleagues reported, in 1958, that the oxidation of α-ketoglutarate and pyruvate in liver homogenates was inhibited by as much as 95 per cent. Moreover, this inhibition could be reversed by the addition of NAD^+, suggesting that the toxin was in some way interfering with the specific NAD^+-dependent dehydrogenases. The enzymes in question are located in the mitochondria and attention was switched, therefore, to the effects of murine toxin on whole mitochondria. The results obtained from these studies seemed to confirm emphatically that the mitochondrion is the site of action of murine toxin. While murine toxin inhibits respiration in intact mitochondria isolated from rat or mouse heart tissue, it has no effect on mitochondria from animal species resistant to the toxin. This led to a belief that murine toxin causes death by inducing heart malfunction, leading to circulatory failure. Attempts to elucidate the molecular mechanism of toxin action revealed that disrupted mitochondria from otherwise resistant animals were susceptible to the action of murine toxin. This confirmed that the toxin acted upon a component located within the mitochondrion. It was finally demonstrated, in 1966, that the toxin inhibits electron transport by blocking NADH-CoQ reductase activity.

Showing that murine toxin inhibits respiration in mitochondria of susceptible animals by blocking NADH-CoQ reductase does not in itself represent unequivocal proof of the mode of action of the toxin *in vivo*, however. To inhibit respiration, the toxin must enter the cell and then enter the mitochondria. Since there is no evidence that the toxin can itself cross the cell membrane, damage to the cell must occur before entry of murine toxin, and thus any effects of the toxin on mitochondria would, for such cells, be secondary and perhaps unimportant *sequelae* to cell membrane damage, a point raised in Chapter 3 in connection with *Clostridium perfringens* α-toxin. Moreover, the amounts of toxin required to inhibit respiration in intact mitochondria are many times greater than those needed to kill a mouse, arguing against mitochondrial damage as the primary pathological lesion induced by the toxin *in vivo*.

More recently, studies using highly purified murine toxin have suggested an alternative mechanism for the action of the toxin. Susceptibility to murine toxin is significantly decreased when mice are fasted, made diabetic, or exposed to an ambient temperature of 37°C. However, susceptibility is increased in mice receiving a high carbohydrate, fat-free diet and exposed to low temperatures. These results suggest that susceptibility is related to the mobilization and metabolism of lipid to glucose, since free fatty acid is preferentially oxidized in fasted or diabetic animals, whereas glucose is preferentially oxidized in mice receiving a high carbohydrate, fat-free diet.

Low temperature increases blockage of free fatty acid mobilization, so animals kept under such conditions would, according to this hypothesis, be expected to be more susceptible to murine toxin. Blockage of lipid mobilization would lead to a drop in blood glucose levels and hypothermia would be the primary cause of death. Certainly, hypothermia has been reported in intoxicated animals and in experimental infection with *Y. pestis*, and it is interesting that mice kept at 37°C are more resistant to the toxin. However, this work, although intriguing, is still in its infancy. Furthermore, despite the large sums of money that have been invested in the study of plague murine toxin, one should not lose sight of the fact that all larger animals, and therefore maybe man, are highly resistant to the toxin, but highly susceptible to *Y. pestis*. Thus, the significance of the toxin in the pathogenesis of human plague must be in considerable doubt.

Guinea pig toxin During the late 1950s and early 1960s, while much effort was directed in the United States towards plague murine toxin, Smith and Keppie were investigating an apparent paradox of *Y. pestis* pathogenicity, the lack of relationship between the susceptibility of laboratory animals to infection and the so-called toxin. They found that guinea pigs and mice injected with toxic preparations from *Y. pestis* grown *in vivo* and *in vitro* died of shock as a result of a drop in blood pressure. In this respect they resembled mice injected with murine toxin. However, the characteristic oedema associated with murine toxin was absent. This and the resistance of guinea pigs to murine toxin suggested that either guinea pigs are killed by a different toxin or that the murine toxin is a degraded form of the native toxin.

To examine this further, whole organisms were disrupted by ultrasonication and separated into soluble extract and insoluble residue. These fractions were then tested for toxicity in mice and guinea pigs. Mouse toxicity (murine toxin) was located almost exclusively in the soluble extract prepared from cells, but guinea pig toxicity was found in both the extract and the residue. Preliminary studies showed that guinea pig toxin consists of at least two components; one is devoid of mouse toxicity, the other contains high mouse toxicity. However, it seemed unlikely that murine toxin was a component of guinea pig toxin, since the component containing high mouse toxicity could be replaced by the ultrasonicate residue, which possessed little or no mouse toxicity.

Subsequently, the British workers succeeded in solubilizing guinea pig toxin from cell wall material and resolved it into two components, neither of which was murine toxin. These two components are relatively non-toxic to guinea pigs when injected separately, but in combination act synergistically. The components as isolated were mainly protein, but did contain some lipid. Thus it was suggested that the virulence of *Y. pestis* may depend on the combined activities of several potentially toxic factors, both protein and lipopolysaccharide, which may be localized in the organism as structural and functional complexes.

Although this work tells us nothing of the pathogenic mechanisms at work in human plague, it is more relevant to the disease than many of the studies of murine toxin, and it is disappointing to think that during the last 15 years so much effort has been put into identifying a sub-mitochondrial site for murine toxin action, while this potentially more fruitful line of research has been totally ignored.

In summary, the nature of the toxin or toxins of *Y. pestis* and their role in the human disease syndrome are still far from clear. The classical approach to such a problem is to prepare a specific toxoid and to determine whether injection of this confers immunity to the disease. Needless to say, the severity of human plague renders such experiments impossible. Until such questions can be answered, however, we are left to argue whether, in the context of plague, man resembles a mouse, monkey or guinea pig.

Summary

Bacterial endotoxin (lipopolysaccharide) is part of the outer layer of the outer membrane of Gram-negative bacteria. It consists of three regions: polysaccharide side chains, which confer sero-specificity; core polysaccharide; and lipid A, which interdigitates into the outer membrane of the bacterium. The toxic properties of endotoxin reside in lipid A and include abortion, pyrogenicity, the Schwartzman reaction, hypotension, shock, and lethality; interaction of endotoxin with granulocytes is presented as being of central importance.

Fever may be caused by direct action on the nervous system or more importantly by interaction of endotoxin with leucocytes and the reticuloendothelial system, stimulating release of an endogenous pyrogen which interacts with the nervous system directly, or *via* prostaglandins. The Schwartzman phenomenon results from endotoxin-induced complement-mediated release of charged proteins from granulocytes which stimulate clotting and vascular coagulation. Hypotension and shock may result either from vascular coagulation or release of histamine, catecholamines or kinins. Lethality is almost certainly the integrated sum of all these effects.

In addition to endotoxin, *Yersinia pestis* produces two other cell-associated toxins: one is only toxic to mice, the other is a complex toxin which consists of at least two synergistic proteins toxic to mice and guinea pigs. The relevance of mouse toxin to experimental plague infection is questionable, while the other toxin reproduces the main features of experimental plague infection in guinea pigs. The role of these toxins in human plague is not known.

References

'Bacterial lipopolysaccharides. The chemistry, biology and clinical significance of endotoxins.' (1973). *J. Inf. Dis. 128*: Supplement No 1.

'Current status and prospects for improved and new bacterial vaccines.' (1977). *J. Inf. Dis. 136*: Supplement. Sections on endotoxin.

EDWARDS, A. J. (1975). 'Ischaemia of the gut.' *Medicine 19*: 909.

HINSHAW, L. B. (1971). 'Release of vasoactive agents and the vascular effects of endotoxin.' In: *Microbial Toxins* Vol. V p. 209. Edited by S. Kadis, G. Weinbaum and S. J. Ajl. Academic Press.

SMITH, H. (1977). 'Microbial surfaces in relation to pathogenicity.' *Bact. Rev. 41*: 475.

SMITH, H. (1960). 'The biochemical response to bacterial injury.' In: *The biochemical response to injury: a symposium organised by the Council for International Organisation of Medical Sciences, established under the joint auspices of UNESCO and WHO p. 341.* Edited by H.B. Stoner and C. J. Threfall. Blackwell Scientific Publications, Oxford.

WALKER, R. V. (1967). 'Plague toxins—a critical review.' *Current topics in microbiology and immunology 41*: 23.

Glossary

Afferent: conducting towards a centre

Antigen: a foreign substance, of high molecular weight, which when introduced into an animal will evoke the production of an antibody.

Antibody: a protein produced by an animal in response to an antigen, that will react specifically with the antigen which triggered its synthesis.

Antitoxin: antibody specific for a toxin

Abomasum: fourth stomach of ruminants

Abomasitis: inflammation of abomasum

Autonomic system: nervous system controlling involuntary muscle movements

Baroreceptors: receptor organ responsive to pressure

Biopsy: examination of tissue removed from the living body.

Cytoskeleton: intracellular structures comprising micro-filaments and micro-tubules whose functions include membrane movement and cell motility.

Caecum: proximal part of the large intestine.

Colitis: inflammation of the colon.

Degranulation: release, by exocytosis, of contents of granules found in white cells.

Efferent: conducting away from a centre

Endocardium: membrane which lines the heart

Endocytosis: uptake by cells of extracellular contents into membrane-bounded vesicles

Endotoxin: lipopolysaccharide component of Gram-negative cell wall

Enterotoxin: toxin synthesized in the lumen of the intestine and whose site of action is the intestinal mucosa

Exocytosis: release by cells of contents of membrane-bounded vesicles or granules

Exotoxin: toxin secreted by organism

Erythema: redness of the skin due to increased blood content

Febrile: feverish

Flaccid: weak, soft, limp

Gastroenteritis: inflammation of stomach and intestines

Granules (in white cells): packets of degradative enzymes which, if released into intracellular vacuoles will digest micro-organisms, and into cell surroundings will damage neighbouring cells

Glomerulus: a small convoluted mass of capillaries such as are found in the functional unit of the kidney

Granulocyte: white cell containing granules

99

Glossary

Granulocytopoenia: depression in the numbers of circulating granulocytes

Granulocytosis: increase in the numbers of circulating granulocytes

Haemoglobinuria: presence of haemoglobin in urine

Haemorrhage: escape of blood from a ruptured vessel

Haemostasis: stoppage of blood flow

HeLa: a much used line of cells of human origin

Hepatosplanchnic: pertaining to the liver and viscera

Humoral: pertaining to fluid; humoral immunity refers to antibody-mediated immunity because antibodies are found in serum and other body fluids

Hydrophilic: 'water-loving' affinity for aqueous environment

Hydrophobic: 'water-hating' affinity for lipids

Hyperaemia: excess blood in a tissue

Hypotension: lowered tension; in particular, low blood pressure

Hypovolaemic: abnormally decreased volume (of blood, for example)

Ileum: the distal portion of the small intestine, ending at the caecum

Immunological response: response of animal to an antigenic stimulus

Immunoglobulin: generic term for antibodies and proteins with same basic structure

Immunity: state of acquired resistance (to a pathogen, for example)

Immunoprecipitate: aggregate of antigen and antibody formed in free solution or in a gel

Infarct: localized area of ischaemic necrosis

Inflammation (inflammatory response): a tissue response to injury, caused by a variety of agents including microbes, characterized by dilatation of blood vessels (hence reddening), exudation of fluid from blood vessels, and infiltration of leucocytes.

Intraepidermal: within the outermost nonvascular (that is, without blood vessels) layer of skin.

***in vitro*:** pertaining to experiments conducted with tissue explants, cultured cells or cell-free extracts outside the intact body.

***in vivo*:** pertaining to experiments conducted in whole animals (or plants).

Ischaemia: local temporary deficiency of blood due to interruption of blood supply

Ligated loop: a section of intact intestine, the lumen of which is sealed at each end by ligatures, left in animal with intact blood and nerve supply.

Leucocyte: general term for all white cells; latter differentiated by size, morphology, staining and function.

Lymphocyte: white cells, involved in immune response

Lymphadenitis: inflammation of lymph nodes

Macrophage: large phagocytic cell

Mesentery: tissue which attaches intestines to the abdominal wall.

Myocardium: muscular substance of the heart

Mitral valve: valve between left auricle and ventricle of the heart

Monocyte: phagocytic white cell

Necrosis: death of cell or tissue caused by some injury

Oedema: abnormal accumulation of fluid in intercellular spaces of the body

Oligaemia: deficiency in volume of blood

Parenchyma: the essential or functional elements of an organ in contrast to its framework

Parenteral: otherwise than through the alimentary canal

Parturient: pertaining to birth

Pathogen: disease-producing organism

Pericardium: membranous sac enclosing the heart

Peritoneum: membrane lining the abdominal wall

Platelets: anucleate cellular components of blood which comprise part of the blood-clotting mechanism

Polymorphonuclear neutrophils: phagocytic granule-containing white cell with multilobed nucleus; differentiated by morphology and staining characteristics.

Portal vein: vessel, carrying blood from intestine to liver

Prophylaxis: prevention of disease

Proventriculus: a pouch at the junction of the foregut and mid gut of insects

Pyogenic: pus-producing

Reticuloendothelial system (RES): phagocytic cells which form a network or 'reticulum' (in spleen and lymph nodes, for example) and line blood vessels or sinuses.

Serous: pertaining to serum

Spore (bacteria): a distinct morphological entity (derived from vegetative cells) capable of extreme longevity and possessing high resistance to chemicals and physical agencies to which vegetative cells are usually susceptible.

Syndrome: a number of concurrent symptoms which constitute a distinct clinical picture

Synaptosome: a preparation rich in nerve endings

Therapy: treatment of disease

Thoracic: pertaining to the chest cavity

Thrombus: a blood clot which forms in a blood vessel and remains at site of origin

Toxoid: detoxified toxin, which will evoke production of antitoxin which will react with original toxin.

Transudation: passage of serum or other fluids through a membrane

Tularaemia: a disease of rodents, transmissible to man, caused by *Yersinia tularensis*

Ungulate: hoofed (animals)

Virulent (a–): highly pathogenic; a–, poorly pathogenic

Viscera: large interior organs, especially those in the abdomen

Index

abortion (see endotoxin)
abrin 34
acetylcholine, inhibition of release by
  botulinum toxin 32
adenylate cyclase
  composition 21
  regulation 21
  stimulation by
    Bacillus cereus enterotoxin 65
    cholera toxin 16
    Escherichia coli heat labile
      enterotoxin 25
    shigella enterotoxin 65
    staphylococcal enterotoxins 63
ADP-ribosylation
  by cholera toxin 20
  by diphtheria toxin 11
  by *Escherischia coli* heat labile
    enterotoxin 25
  by *Pseudomonas aeruginosa* toxins 15
aggressin 7, 59, 78
alpha toxin
  Clostridium bifermentans 46
  C. novyi 10, 44, 58
  C. perfringens 3, 37
  C. septicum 44
  C. sordellii 42
  staphylococcal 50,53
anthrax 59
anthrax toxin 3–4, 60
  discovery 61
  role in disease 62
antitoxin 2, 43
Bacillus
  anthracis 3 (see also anthrax toxin)
  cereus
    cereolysin 47
    diarrhoeagenic toxin 65
    emetic toxin 65
    enterotoxins 65
  subtilis
    subtilysin 49
black disease 73
black quarter 74
botulinum toxin 10–11, 26
  mode of action 29
  structure 28
botulism 2, 27
braxy 74
cereolysin 47
cholera 4, 16

choleragen (see cholera toxin)
choleragenoid 18
cholera toxin (choleragen) 16
  entry mechanism 23
  immunogenicity 24
  mode of action 17
  receptor 21
  structure 18
  subunit A_1 18
  subunit A_2 18
  subunit B 18
  Texas star 24–25
clostridial diseases 71
Clostridium
  bifermentans
    alpha toxin (phospholipase C) 46
  botulinum
    neurotoxin (see botulin toxin)
  chauvoei
    black quarter 74
  difficile
    pseudomembranous colitis 72
  histolyticum 37
    alpha toxin 37
    gas gangrene 36, 41, 44
  novyi
    alpha toxin 10–11, 44, 58
    black disease 73
    gas gangrene 71
    redwater disease 73
  perfringens
    alpha toxin 3, 37
      mode of action 40
      role in infection 41
    beta toxin 72
    enterotoxaemia in sheep 72
    enterotoxin 64
    gas gangrene 37
    lamb dysentery 72
    pig bel 71
    phospholipase C (see alpha toxin)
    theta toxin (perfringolysin) 44, 47, 49
  septicum
    braxy 74, 37, 44
    gas gangrene 3
  tetani 26
    neuroxin (see tetanus toxin)
    tetanolysin 27, 47
colicin
  E2 34
  E3 33

Corynebacterium
  diphtheriae 9
    toxin (see diphtheria toxin)
  ovis 9
  sphingomyelinase D 45
corynephages 9
cross-reacting material, CRM
  CRM_{45} 13–14
  CRM_{197} 13
cyclic AMP 17, 64
diarrhoeagenic toxin, from *Bacillus
  cereus* 65
diphtheria 9
diphtheria toxin 4, 9
  cross-reacting material 9, 13
  cytotoxic activity 11
  entry mechanism 13
  fragment A 12–13
  fragment B 12–13
  inhibition of protein synthesis 4, 11
  receptor 13
  structure 11
  synthesis
    lysogeny 9
    regulation 10
    tox gene 9
dysentery 65
  lamb 72
elongation factor 2 (EF2) 11, 16
emetic toxin, from *Bacillus cereus* 65
endotoxin (lipopolysaccharide) 78
  abortion 81
  hypotension 87
  lethality 92
  location in bacterium 80
  protection with antibody 92
  pyrogenicity 82
  Schwartzman reaction 85
  shock 87
  structure 80
  tolerance 82
  Yersinia pestis 93
enterotoxaemia in sheep 72
enterotoxin 4
  Bacillus cereus 65
  cholera 4, 16
  Clostridium perfringens 64
  Escherichia coli
    heat labile 25
    heat stable 26
  staphylococcal 63
  Vibrio cholerae 4, 16
erythrocytes
  avian, adenylate cyclase 6–7
  and membrane damage 11, 14
Escherichia coli
  colicin E2 34
  colicin E3 33
  enterotoxin
    heat labile (LT) 25
    heat stable (ST) 26
    role in pathogenesis 26

exfoliatin 68
exotoxin A, *Pseudomonas aeruginosa* 15
food poisoning
  Bacillus cereus 65
  botulism 27
  Clostridium perfringens
    type A 64
    type C 64
  staphylococcal 63
fragment A
  abrin 34
  botulinum toxin 28
  diphtheria toxin 12–13
  ricin 34
  tetanus toxin 28
fragment B
  abrin 34
  botulinum toxin 28
  diphtheria toxin 12–13
  ricin 34
  tetanus toxin 28
gamma-amino butyric acid (GABA),
  inhibition of release by tetanus toxin 30
ganglioside, and
  botulinum toxin 32
  cholera toxin 19
  tetanus toxin 31
  GM_1 19
gas gangrene 3, 37, 71
glycine, inhibition of release by tetanus
  toxin 30
glycoprotein hormones 34
GTP hydrolysis, inhibition by,
  abrin 34
  cholera toxin 21
  ricin 34
guanylate cyclase, stimulation by
  Escherichia coli heat stable enterotoxin 26
guinea pig toxin, *Yersinia pestis* 96
haemolysis, hot-cold 40, 46
hypersensitivity 1
hypotension (see endotoxin)
immunopathological damage 1
infant botulism 27
lamb dysentery 72
lecithinase (see phospholipase C)
lectin 34
leucocidin, staphylococcal 51
lipid A 80
lipopolysaccharide (see endotoxin)
lysogeny, and toxigenicity 9
mastitis 55
membrane
  constituents 5
  structure 5
membrane damaging toxins 36
murine toxin, *Yersinia pestis* 95
neurotoxin
  botulinum toxin 27
  shigella enterotoxin 65
  staphylococcal enterotoxins 63
  tetanus toxin 27

neurotransmission, inhibition by
  botulinum and tetanus toxins 32
Panton-Valentine leucocidin 51
perfringolysin
  see *Clostridium perfringens* θ toxin 47
phosphatidyl choline 3, 40
phospholipases 5, 40
phospholipase C
  Clostridium bifermentans 46
  Clostridium perfringens (alpha toxin) 3, 40
phosphoryl choline 3
pig bel 71
plague 93
  toxins, see *Yersinia pestis*
plasmids and toxigenicity 11
prostaglandins 83
protein A, of colicin E3 34
protein synthesis, inhibition by
  abrin 34
  colicin E3 33
  diphtheria toxin 4, 11
  Pseudomonas aeruginosa exotoxin A 15
  ricin 34
pseudomembranous colitis 72
Pseudomonas aeruginosa
  exoenzyme S 16
  exotoxin A 15
pyrogen, endogenous 82
pyrogenicity (see endotoxin)
receptor
  cholera toxin 21
  diphtheria toxin 13
  shigella enterotoxin 67
redwater disease 73
reticulo-endothelial system, and
  endotoxin 83
ricin 34
Schwartzman reaction (see endotoxin)
Shigella
  dysenteriae type 1 65
  enterotoxins 67
shock (see endotoxin)
sphingomyelinase D, *Corynebacterium
  ovis* 45
staphylococcal scalded skin syndrome
  (SSSS) 68
staphylococcal toxins
  alpha toxin 50
    role in infection 53
  beta-haemolysin 45, 46
  delta toxin 49
    synergy with alpha toxin 57
  enterotoxins 63

exfoliatin 11, 68
gamma toxin 51
leucocidin (Panton-Valentine) 51
  role in infection 53
streptococcal toxins 10–11, 75
  erythrogenic toxin
    potentiation of streptolysin-O and
      endotoxin 76
  streptolysin-O
    mode of action 48
    role in disease 48
  streptolysin-S 57
streptolysin-O 48
streptolysin-S 57
subtilysin 49
sub-unit toxins 9
surfactant toxins 49
synergy between,
  different toxins (same organism) 57
  different toxins (separate organism) 76
  toxic factors
    anthrax toxin 61
    guinea pig plague toxin 97
    staphylococcal γ-haemolysin 51
    staphylococcal leucocidin 51
TEN, (see toxic epidermal necrolysis)
tetanolysin 27, 47
tetanospasmin, (see tetanus toxin)
tetanus 26
tetanus toxin (tetanospasmin)
  mode of action 29
  structure 28
  transport 31
theta toxin, *Clostridium perfringens* 44, 49
thiol-activated cytolysins 37, 46
  activation 47
  mode of action 48
  role in disease 48
tolerance, (see endotoxin)
tox gene, diphtheria toxin 9
toxic epidermal necrolysis (TEN) 68
toxin, definition 7
toxoid 2
triphosphoinositide, and staphylococcal
  leucocidin 52
tuberculin 2
Ussing chamber 17
Vibrio cholerae 4, 16
  enterotoxin, (see Cholera toxin)
Yersinia pestis toxins 93
  endotoxin 94
  guinea pig toxin 96
  murine toxin 95